Ethics, Medicine, and Information Technology

Ethics, Medicine, and Information Technology

Intelligent Machines and the Transformation of Health Care

Kenneth W. Goodman

Professor and Director, University of Miami Miller School of Medicine Institute for Bioethics and Health Policy, Miami, FL, USA

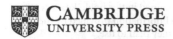
CAMBRIDGE
UNIVERSITY PRESS

CAMBRIDGE
UNIVERSITY PRESS

University Printing House, Cambridge CB2 8BS, United Kingdom

One Liberty Plaza, 20th Floor, New York, NY 10006, USA

477 Williamstown Road, Port Melbourne, VIC 3207, Australia

314-321, 3rd Floor, Plot 3, Splendor Forum, Jasola District Centre, New Delhi - 110025, India

79 Anson Road, #06-04/06, Singapore 079906

Cambridge University Press is part of the University of Cambridge.

It furthers the University's mission by disseminating knowledge in the pursuit of education, learning and research at the highest international levels of excellence.

www.cambridge.org
Information on this title: www.cambridge.org/9781107624733

First published 2015

A catalogue record for this publication is available from the British Library

Library of Congress Cataloging in Publication data
Goodman, Kenneth W., 1954– , author.
Ethics, medicine, and information technology : intelligent machines
and the transformation of health care / Kenneth W. Goodman.
    p. ; cm.
Includes bibliographical references and index.
ISBN 978-1-107-62473-3 (paperback)
I. Title. [DNLM: 1. Medical Informatics Applications.
2. Biomedical Research – ethics. 3. Confidentiality – ethics. 4. Electronic Health
Records – ethics. 5. Telemedicine – ethics. W 26.5]
R858
610.285–dc23

2015012826

ISBN 978-1-107-62473-3 Paperback

Contents

Preface and acknowledgments

The intersection of ethics, computing, and the health professions was rather small nearly two decades ago when an edited volume attempted to plot it (Goodman 1998a). That book seemed to meet and stimulate a need. The subsequent dizzying growth of health information technology, or biomedical informatics, was an evolution from an interesting curiosity to a new professional field at the center of nearly everything in the health professions, and the ethical issues it raised emerged as essential for professional practice, education, and public policy. The present volume tries to identify and address the most significant of those issues.

The field of bioethics, itself also quite young, had been fledged on the introduction of new technologies in clinical care and research. Linking bioethics anew to informatics seemed to be both an opportunity and an obligation.

This book is written for clinicians, researchers, and students who work in health information technology and have an interest in ethics, and for ethics professionals and students who have come to realize the importance and scope of such technology. Only a basic knowledge of the fields forming the intersection is required. I try throughout to introduce useful ethical concepts in such a way as to invite and guide clinicians and scientists without disappointing bioethics experts. Policy makers will also find either something useful or something to be angry about. If any thought, conversation, or improved policy is thereby stimulated, the anger will have been worthwhile.

The eight chapters, enumerated and briefly introduced in Chapter 1, seemed natural subdivisions of our three-way intersection, though it certainly would have been possible to have identified different seams and demarcations. Although a Venn diagram plotting the three fields would be simple enough, different subdivisions are also possible. In addition, some issues demand to be revisited in different places; so Chapter 3, on privacy and confidentiality, must lend some of its content to Chapter 8, on research.

It is a source of some wonderment that the world's bioethics community has not made more hay of health information technology. We enjoy extensive literatures on genetics and ethics, neuroethics, nanoethics, and so on, but there is little comparable when it comes to biomedical informatics. Fortunately, that is changing. A major bioethics journal, *The Cambridge Quarterly of Healthcare Ethics*, now features a section on health information technology (which I edit thanks to the encouragement, gentle suasion, and support of Tomi Kushner); and, as the list of references in this book makes clear, interest in ethics and informatics is increasing across several intellectual divides. If I am right about the scope and importance of ethics and informatics, this is very good news.

To write a book is to incur many debts, and, in this case, all gladly. Several grants have supported the work here. Thus:

- Work on this book was supported by the University of Miami CTSI, funded by the National Center for Advancing Translational Sciences at the National Institutes of Health, grant #1UL1TR000460.
- The discussion of personal health records was supported by a grant from the Robert Wood Johnson Foundation to Project HealthDesign.

- This work was also supported in part by the Center for Law, Ethics and Applied Research in Health Information (CLEAR; http://clearhealthinfo.iu.edu) at Indiana University, which grants permission for its use in this book.
- Some of the discussion of end-of-life care and its representation in the electronic health record was supported by a grant to the University of Florida and the University of Miami by the Alpha-1 Foundation.
- Philanthropist Adrienne Arsht has provided unparalleled support and encouragement.

The University of Miami has been a supportive and congenial home for such multi- and interdisciplinary work, and I acknowledge several colleagues in the chapters here: I want to signal special thanks to Richard Bookman, Robin N. Fiore, and Joanna Johnson, variously, for support, guidance, encouragement, muse-like assistance, and improvement of the manuscript. Students and faculty at the University of Miami Miller School of Medicine have both endured exposure to some of the material herein and improved it. Ana Bezanilla, Gigi Giobio, and Sara Charles of the school's Institute for Bioethics and Health Policy provided first-rate bibliographic and related support.

I have been fortunate to enjoy the support of a number of organizations and, especially, the people who comprise them. AMIA (formerly the American Medical Informatics Association) has been an intellectual home for more than two decades, supporting the creation of an ethics working group, including ethics in conference programming, featuring ethics in its journal, and taking the counsel of members who include bioethics in their areas of competence and expertise. Election as a Fellow of the American College of Medical Informatics has conferred such recognition that I am convinced it was a mistake. I have enjoyed the friendship, mentorship, and encouragement of several AMIA leaders, including Randy Miller, Ted Shortliffe, Chuck Jaffe, Patti Brennan, Eta Berner, Bill Tierney, and Don Detmer.

Versions and aspects of material from several chapters have been shared and bettered during formal presentations at a number of institutions in addition to several talks at the University of Miami: the American College of Epidemiology, European National Ethics Councils Forum, Fundación Santa Fe of Bogotá, Health Level Seven (HL7), Indiana University School of Medicine, Johns Hopkins University Division of Health Sciences Informatics, New Jersey Medical School, New York University Center for Health Informatics & Bioinformatics, University of Florida College of Medicine, University of Texas Health Sciences Center, the US Food and Drug Administration, and the World Health Organization. Obviously, none of these institutions has endorsed or is in any way responsible for the contents here.

I have tried throughout the book to provide historical context, and, for Chapter 1, for instance, this led me to enjoy the hospitality of, and now extend thanks to, Alice Stevenson, Curator at University College London's Petrie Museum of Egyptian Archaeology, who arranged for me to view the "Kahun Medical Papyrus" there, the oldest known medical record.

I am deeply grateful to my wife, Jackie Schneider, who evinced plenary and Olympian patience and provided inestimable help with the manuscript, and my daughter, Allison Goodman, for reminding me why we do things like write books and that, when one has said enough, one should stop.

Information technologies and twenty-first-century clinical practice

Ethics and the electronic health record

The slow death of maintaining patient records on paper has precipitated a new era. Electronic health records are now required. This is not about fashion, the designs of regulators, or the ambitions of administrators. These electronic records are required because the paper chart was a terrible way to store and (try to) retrieve patient information. It harmed patients. As we will see here, electronic records, in conjunction with personal health records, are transforming the health information ecosystem. This transformation presents us with an ensemble of interesting and important ethical issues, a review of which serves as an introduction to this volume.

Bioethics and health information technology

More than genetics and stem cells, more than left-ventricular-assist devices and extra-corporeal membrane oxygenation, more than organ transplants and gamma knives and nanomedicine and ovarian hyperstimulation – more than any technology of the sort that tends to raise or contribute to interesting and difficult ethical issues – it is the use of computers and communication technologies that will affect the lives of people in the twenty-first century. In the other direction, more human lives will be touched by health information technology than any other technology, ever.

The history of bioethics is in many respects the history of our coming to terms with technology. The machines, tools, and processes that have defined modern health care also press against moral intuitions about the beginning of life, the end of life, and the sometimes rocky journey in the middle. Bioethics 101 is, at least in part, about whether a tool should be used; if so, when and by whom; and, then, by what lights, guidelines, principles, or rules. Most of these tools and technologies help us to see or hear better and to touch or cut with greater sensitivity or precision. They help us to rescue our very cells, clean them, move them, numb them, change them, or kill them; nowadays we even make them.

The tools of information technology are different: These machines can *think* for us. The processes or functions they assist include cognition, reason, and memory.

Medical books and other texts do this too, to some extent, sometimes. But a book (or papyrus scroll or Web page) is, for our purposes here, best thought of as a repository. A book can hold the facts we are looking for, though an e-book can readily be searched; it can help us learn, though the practices of medicine or nursing will never adequately be learned by reading alone; and it can help teach us to reason, but not reason for us. The change from paper-based health records to electronic records is as transformational as the transition from illuminated manuscripts to moveable type was – perhaps greater. The availability of computer decision support systems makes plain the fact that intelligent machines have inferential and analytic powers that likely exceed those of humans. The ability of computers and associated telecommunications tools to collect, store, and transmit information can turn every clinical encounter into a research event and help fuel a cyclone of science.

The electronic health record, conceived as the successor to the ancient system of keeping records on paper and intended to keep track of health and medical data for patients, emerges as a research tool, embeds decision support systems, enables analyses for quality and resource allocation, and, generally, transforms the way health and medical information are collected and used. Electronic health records cost fortunes and should be able to help coordinate the care of people who are sick and dying. It would be good if we got it right. That has unfortunately turned out to be quite difficult.

What health records are for

The oldest known medical records are contained in the Kahun Papyrus. Dating from Egypt's Middle Kingdom, it is about 3,800 years old and deals mostly with women's health, obstetrics, and gynecology. Mostly, it gives advice. In this respect, this papyrus scroll therefore likely contains the first practice guidelines. It contains 34 prescriptions and instructions for addressing sterility, managing childbirth, and attempting contraception. The prescriptions reveal a diverse pharmacopeia, including the use of herbs, beer, milk, oil, dates, incense, and crocodile dung, which is to be chopped, combined with sour milk, and burned, apparently for a woman to stand over as a contraceptive (Smith 2013). A different translation suggests that the crocodile dung should be placed in a pessary and positioned "at the mouth of her womb" (Stevens 1975, 931).[1] Another recipe calls for honey to be sprinkled on the woman, who should be on a bed of natron, or carbonate salt (Smith 2011); or that the natron should be added to honey and then inserted in the vagina (Stevens 1975). It is not clear precisely when this application should occur or, indeed, how long it would last. Another honey-based, intravaginal contraceptive is said to work for "one, two or three years" (ibid.). While these might be the first practice guidelines, it is clear they are not to be regarded as evidence based.

Now visit the Web site http://archive.nlm.nih.gov/proj/ttp/books.htm and click around. The "Turning the Pages Information System" was originally created by the British Library, and it has been adopted and adapted by the US National Library of Medicine "for visitors to touch and turn the pages of virtual books." The first "book" on display has come to be known as "The Edwin Smith Surgical Papyrus" (Al-Awqati 2006; Gillum 2013). Here is Case 22, about fractures of the temporal bone:

> If you treat a man for a fracture in his temple, you have to put your finger on his chin and your finger on the end of his ramus [of the mandible]. Blood will fall from his nostrils and the interior of his ears from that fracture. Wipe for him with a plug of cloth until you see its [bone] chips inside his ears. If you have called to him and he is dazed and does not speak, then you say about him, "One who has a fracture in his temple, who bleeds from his nostrils and his ears, is dazed and suffers stiffness in his neck: an ailment for which nothing is done."
>
> (Al-Awqati 2006, 2114)

This is perhaps the first documented case of clinical futility. Al-Awqati writes, "the conclusions remain correct to this day" (ibid.).

This is a case study, a guideline, and a teaching tool. These early attempts to record what healers encountered and to share with others are the first-known intellectual and conceptual antecedents of today's electronic health records. By the time of Hippocrates more than a millennium later, case studies had become common, and were still used to teach. While the historical Hippocrates is actually elusive and vague, the case histories attributed to him are early masterpieces of observation and documentation, and they fueled the inchoate sciences of diagnosis and prognosis. When Hippocrates and his students got it right, it was in part because they learned from previous patients. As we will see in Chapter 8, the ancient use of one patient's information to try to help another patient is near the foundation of obligations to make de-identified health care information available for research and other legitimate analysis, sometimes without the consent of those who are the sources of the information.

The Hippocratic case report is chronological, sometimes blunt: "Thirty-fourth day. Death" (Reiser 1991, 902). The chronological structure supported the Greeks' interest in what Reiser calls "therapeutic timing" and on symptoms "most predictive of outcome. The Hippocratic physician used this prognostic power to decide which cases to accept or decline. This action had its origin in a fundamental tenet of Greek medicine of this period, namely, that futile therapy should not be used" (ibid.).[2]

The seventeenth-century physician Thomas Sydenham (1624–1689), called by some the "English Hippocrates," likewise saw patterns in the symptoms reported by his patients and elicited from these patterns distinctive profiles of diseases. Reiser attributes this in part to Sydenham's work at the dawn of the age of classification of plants and animals (Linnaeus published his *Philosophia Botanica* in 1751 and the *Species Plantarum* in 1753), and it inspired in him the ability to "synthesize from clinical records the case histories of individual patients into a disease history" (ibid., 903). These disease histories were of the greatest ontological significance: Diseases emerged as entities with specific etiologies and distinctive properties. This insight is the conceptual antecedent of contemporary work in biomedical ontology[3] and undergirds work in computational genomics and work on the Semantic Web. It is the great-grandparent of The International Classification of Diseases (e.g., ICD-9 and ICD-10) maintained by the World Health Organization; ICD codes undergird some computerized decision support systems and medical billing protocols.

Where Sydenham's case histories emphasized patients' self-reports, the French physician René Laennec (1781–1826) flipped the medical record to highlight physicians' observations and measurements. He was inspired in part by modesty: Where physicians since antiquity had listened to hearts by placing their ears on patients' chests, Laennec regarded the practice with female patients as "conduct unbecoming to the gentleman doctor" (ibid., 904). He placed a rolled tube of paper on a patient's chest and found that heart sounds traveled clearly through the tube. This invention, the stethoscope, enabled more precise auscultation and hence fostered a flow of increasingly reliable data into the case report. Listen:

> A man, aged 65, came into hospital on the 29th of November [apparently 1819], affected with slight pulmonary symptoms, chiefly marked by dyspnea, to which he had been long subject, and which he considered as Asthma. Percussion afforded no result, owing to the excessive fatness of the individual; only the chest appeared to sound somewhat less below the right clavicle. Respiration was inaudible over the whole of the right side, but was very sonorous on the left. From these results I considered this person as affected with a latent peripneumony [pneumonia] of the right lung.
>
> Five days after this, there was observed slight oedema of the right side of the chest; and on applying the stethoscope to the back, respiration was somewhat perceptible along the edge of the spine on the right side, though less so than on the left. There was very little

cough, and scarcely any expectoration. These symptoms indicating pleurisy rather than peripneumony, necessarily modified our diagnostics. After a few days the oppression became less, and we began to hear the sound of respiration, in a slight degree, below the right clavicle ... On the eleventh [day] the chest sounded still better in this point, and respiration became distinct as in the opposite side, but was not perceptible lower than the third rib. It was, also, sufficiently distinct between the spine and scapula. At this time the patient expectorated some opaque, yellow, puriform [purulent] sputa. The symptoms continued much the same until the middle of February, when he died, apparently from an attack of peritonitis. (Laennec 1821, 398–9; cf. Reiser 1991)

The information contained in the medical record forms the basis for diagnosis. It is a story, but a story made useful by efforts at precision and rigor, efforts embodied in the medical record. Alas, available treatments lagged, and at the time the best response to tuberculosis, for instance, involved the application of leeches.

At about the same time in North America, David Hosack (the physician who unsuccessfully attended to former US secretary of the treasury Alexander Hamilton in his duel with Vice President Aaron Burr in 1804) suggested that some cases were especially good for teaching medical students, and so should be carefully recorded. The Board of Governors of the Society of the New York Hospital had already approved the first hospital rules, in 1793, such that the "apothecary prepared and delivered a monthly report of the 'Names and Diseases of the Persons, received, deceased or discharged in the same, with the date of each event, and the Place from whence the Patients last came'" (Siegler 2010, 672). In 1805, the board agreed with Dr. Hosack: "The house-physician, with the aid of his assistant, under the direction of the attending physician, shall keep a register of all medical cases which occur in the hospital, and which the latter shall think worthy of preservation, which book shall be neatly bound, and kept in the library for the inspection of the friends of the patients, the governors, physicians and surgeons, and the students attending the hospital" (ibid.). By 1830, it was required that all cases be recorded and that no one could be appointed a House Physician or Surgeon until he had entered at least 12 cases in the register.

The history and evolving utility of the medical record intersect at interesting points with the history of evidence-based practice. Good case records can help evaluate the effectiveness of therapies. Perhaps the first instance of this was the discovery that the long-standing practice of bloodletting did not work. Bloodletting, a consequence of the humoral theory of disease, had been practiced since antiquity in several cultures. It was responsible for countless deaths (including perhaps that of George Washington, who died after some five pints of blood were removed by his doctors [Morens 1999]). The French physician Pierre Charles Alexandre Louis (1787–1872) undertook a detailed review of hospital cases and determined by a simple analysis, which he called the "numerical method," that bloodletting was by no means curative and, on the contrary, generally harmful (Louis 1836; cf. Louis 1835). Earlier he had written:

As to different methods of treatment, it is possible for us to assure ourselves of the superiority of one or other ... by enquiring if the greater number of individuals have been cured by one means than another. Here it is necessary to count. And it is, in great part at least, because hitherto this method has not at all, or rarely been employed, that the science of therapeutics is so uncertain. (Louis 1834, 26–28)[4]

This numerical method has been cited as a significant milestone in the history of evidence-based practice (Sackett et al. 2000; cf. Goodman 2003), despite flaws in some analyses.[5]

The nineteenth and twentieth centuries saw sustained use of the hospital record in medical education. In 1910, Massachusetts General Hospital began weekly conferences to review cases and analyze "clinical logic" of patient management (comparing clinical and pathologic analyses); in 1915 the hospital began publishing the cases and analyses for subscribers, prompting one physician to write, "To a great many of us, these cases are the only postgraduate work we have at the present time" (Reiser 1991, 907). By 1923, case studies and analyses had become a regular feature of the *Boston Medical and Surgical Journal*. Even after the journal was renamed in 1928, and to the present day, "Case Records of the Massachusetts General Hospital" remains a weekly feature of *The New England Journal of Medicine*.

The medical record increased in formality with a commensurate loss in narrative. "House physicians," writes Siegler, "no longer summarized the course of a patient's hospitalization; they recorded their observations but not their thinking" (Siegler 2010, 675).

The need for careful documentation was magnified by social factors and movements. The United Kingdom's National Insurance Act of 1911 required health insurance for workers and that participating general practitioners keep medical records in a specific format, in part to ensure that useful health information about workers could be analyzed. This initiative was put on hold as a wartime measure in 1917; a postwar commission tried to stipulate what information should be contained in the records. This is what it came up with, in part as an inducement to improve the quality of care: "We consider, therefore, that on the whole the most advantageous system will be to require such notes to be kept for every case treated as are likely to be of value to the practitioner himself, or to any other practitioner treating the same patient in subsequent illnesses; and we recommend that the obligations be thus defined" (Tait 1981, 703). This could be said to be patient-centered, though in the ensuing decades difficulties arose in the size of the envelope used to hold the forms – largely because the size of the envelope was stipulated to fit the metal file cabinets already in use (ibid.). Difficulties continued through the creation of the National Health Service in 1946; one reformer in the 1970s noted the absence of a place to record important background information.

The inevitable move from a paper record to an electronic one – some hospitals still have not completed it – exemplifies the way change often occurs in applied sciences such as medicine: There was no experiment, no vote, no edict. Some partisans, activists, and forward-lookers simply began the process of development and adoption. It is a primitive approach, but it has worked well enough often enough to invite tolerance, if not command enthusiasm. It is an embodiment of the anonymous quip, "Modern man is just ancient man – with way better electronics."

What is right – and wrong – with electronic health records

In an early and important attempt to identify and address ethical issues raised by electronic health records (EHR), the philosopher Eike-Henner Kluge suggests that the primary difference between paper and electronics "lies in their logical natures as records and the functional manipulations to which they can be subjected. For instance, electronic patient records can be manipulated in a holistic fashion to yield an integrated picture (representation) of the patient which can be directly involved in, and integrated into, the decision-making process that surrounds patients and health care consumers in a way that is not possible for paper-based records" (2001, 20). It has developed that Professor Kluge was optimistic and so limned a state of affairs that is more aspirational than descriptive. Electronic records *should* have a structure that permits such integration – but, as it develops, they do not. Worse, and as we will see in Chapter 5, the uncontroversially worthy goal of interoperability remains outside our grasp.

That electronic records must replace paper ones is not seriously in dispute. Paper records are "woefully inadequate for meeting the needs of modern medicine" (Shortliffe and Blois 2014, 5). They are inefficient, difficult to read, counterintuitive, cumbersome, difficult to correct meaningfully, and give up their information reluctantly if at all – sifting through large sheaves of paper to acquire important information about a patient is a fool's errand, a frustrating, dispiriting, and sometimes quixotic exercise. Indeed, we have known this for a very long time, at least in some respects (Whiting-O'Keefe et al. 1985). The history of paper (and papyrus) records notwithstanding, they have lost their capacity to save and help recover facts, as well as their ability to deliver patient narratives.

Obligations to improve electronic records

Electronic records are rich in facts, often redundantly, and they, too, do no honor to patient stories. The literature of complaints about, shortcomings in, and failures of electronic records has become a growth industry (just for instance: Bernat 2013; DeAngelis 2014; Hill et al. 2013; Koppel et al. 2005). Wears (2015) despairs for the future of electronic health records, and notes the development of the "shadow chart" to fill gaps in existing systems (Wears 2008). There remain serious questions about the history and course of England's national program for health information technology (Greenhalgh and Keen 2013), alleged to be a source of "patient harm or death" (Magrabi et al. 2015). Many, if not most, of these criticisms are smart, concerned, and constructive. There is much room for improvement, both in the behavior of electronic record users (Chapter 4) and in system manufacture and oversight (Chapters 5 and 6). Between dark nihilism and slavish boosterism lies a sober middle ground, a position that simultaneously recognizes electronic health records as both irreplaceable and improvable; we want to be able to move toward a kind of "electronic standard of care" to which all would aspire and, indeed, would meet. This points to the first of several ethical challenges and, especially, simple-to-state and interlocking ethical obligations (EO):

Improve electronic health records. (EO 1)

In many respects, other chapters in this volume address ways in which such improvement might occur: electronic records must foster reliable decision support, be secure and protect privacy, be used appropriately by well-trained professionals, be safe and interoperable, be patient-centered and manufactured and sold as such, and support research and public health. There is a great deal of work to be done. Such work has, indeed, begun in the form of measured and thoughtful analyses of EHR functions, use, and utility (Kuhn et al. 2015; Mamykina et al. 2012).

Consider the Ebola scare of 2014 and, especially, the allegation that a hospital's electronic health record either did not have the information that a patient (i) presented with fever, dizziness, nausea, abdominal pain, a sharp headache, and decreased urination, and (ii) was from Liberia; or did have the information but was unable to link or synthesize it for clinicians (Upadhyay et al. 2014). We need to collect and study case studies of systems working well, and of systems behaving badly; of humans using tools correctly, or dimly; and so on. Such cases, reviews, analyses, and assays are essential to establish an evidence-base to guide and inform improvement. This entails a second duty:

Expand research on electronic health records. (EO 2)

Such research ought not only to find out what is wrong, but identify best practices. For instance, a common complaint about electronic records, namely their intrusiveness in the clinical encounter (Lown and Rodriguez 2012), should inspire us to explore and document ways to reduce and manage that intrusiveness. In response to the apparent need to type and click during patient encounters, some clinicians have come to share documentation duties with patients, even turning the screen so patients can see what is being entered and so have the opportunity to add, correct, or question.[6] Such a practice can even help improve patients' digital health literacy, itself a worthy topic of research. Some of these issues are taken up in Chapter 4.

There has been a sea change over the past quarter-century in the relationship between patients and their information (we will expand on this shortly, in a review of personal health records). Because patients want and ought to have access to their information (Patel et al. 2014), we must do a better job of respecting that desire and facilitating that access. Generally speaking, and all other things being equal, there is no good reason not to allow patients to see their records, to share them, to make them available for research and analysis, and, indeed, to exercise control over access to their records. (Privacy law in the United States, for instance, requires that patients be able to review their records but makes an exception for psychotherapy notes; this is not unreasonable.) The "Blue Button" utility for online patient portals, developed by the US Department of Veterans Affairs as part of its personal health record system, is a splendid example of efforts to reduce or eliminate barriers to patient access to their information (Turvey et al. 2014), and to share it for health service research (Nazi et al. 2010). Furthermore, it has been widely and compellingly suggested that patients should also enjoy "granular control" over those who view their information, and, moreover, such a feature of EHR design can be driven by adherence to various principles of bioethics (Meslin et al. 2013; Meslin and Schwartz 2014). This celebration of applied autonomy or functional self-determination suggests a third obligation to be met in the ongoing improvement of electronic health records:

Foster and support patient access to and control of their information. (EO 3)

In the next chapter, on computerized decision support, we will emphasize the importance of system evaluation, especially in the contexts in which systems will be used. The long-standing advice to conduct such evaluation seems rarely to be taken. This is also true of research, findings in human factors science, and studies related to organizational and social issues. This points to a divide, a disconnect, between the development and manufacture of electronic health records, on the one hand, and human factors science (e.g., Lowry et al. 2015), and organizational issues, on the other (e.g., Kaplan and Shaw 2004). It might even be safe to infer that if such considerations were given greater weight, electronic health record systems would function better. This suggests a fourth duty:

Improve usability by addressing and accommodating human factors, social and organizational issues, and system research. (EO 4)

Indeed, and as a result of many causes, systems suffer from poor usability, and this has itself assumed a central role in debates over the status and future of electronic health records. Usability issues may be regarded as central to many of the challenges we address in this book, perhaps especially including safety (see Chapter 5). Concerns about unintended consequences of EHR design and implementation have led to a variety of attempts to recommend system improvements.

The Institute of Medicine's 2012 report, *Health IT and Patient Safety: Building Safer Systems for Better Care*, made nine applicable recommendations; Middleton and others (2013) recommend 14 "usability principles"; and the American Medical Association identifies a suite of eight "priorities to improve electronic health record usability" (American Medical Association 2014). Note the similarities between some of these principles and priorities and several of the ethical obligations being identified here.[7]

Personal health records

If you are old enough, you might have had the experience of being informed that you may not look at or have a copy of your medical record. "It's a *medical* record," I was once told, impatiently and incredulously. Her brow was knitted and her mouth opened, literally slack-jawed. This is what she meant:

1. They are notes made by a licensed physician who intended they be used to jog his memory and to share with other physicians as needed.
2. These pages were simply and utterly not to be shared with me, the patient, who had done something outré and improper by asking to take a look.
3. If I was moving to another city, I could not be entrusted to deliver a copy of my medical record to my new physician – that new physician would have to send a letter requesting my chart, which would then be sent directly, doctor to doctor.

The medical record was special, and so, special anointment was required for access. Moreover, it was not exactly clear what use or interest a patient might have in this special collection of Latin abbreviations, hard-to-read observations, and authoritative diagnostic scrawls. This was the age, recall, of hard-to-read prescriptions (sometimes joked about) and occult runes: privileged, secret, and not for you. Moreover, a patient might draw the wrong conclusion, and sharing the record might even be atherapeutic.

As we saw just earlier, however, there is no good reason to prohibit patient access to the records kept of their clinical and hospital history and treatments. Moreover, patients do not want merely to access and to some extent control use of their health information – they also want a role in tracking and generating or producing it. Patients know more than reckoned, and this can likely be put to good use – for them. Consider:

- According to University of Wisconsin Professor Patricia Flatley Brennan, National Program Director for the Robert Wood Johnson Foundation's Project HealthDesign: "Doctors and nurses are experts in clinical care; patients are experts in their daily experiences. Both need to share more with each other and health data from everyday life can help bridge that gap."[8]
- "'This patient knows more about her disease than I do.' This passing remark was made more than 30 years ago to a group of new medical students as we stood around the bedside of a woman with long-standing diabetes mellitus. It is a sentiment that has probably been expressed or felt by doctors many thousands of times since ... Yet until

recently the wisdom and experience of the patient has been only a tacit form of knowledge whose potential to improve the outcome of care and quality of life has been largely untapped. In England alone, there are now nearly 10 million people with a chronic disease. It has been estimated that non-communicable diseases account for almost 40% of deaths in developing countries and 75% in industrialised countries" (Donaldson 2003, commenting on a chronic disease self-management program).

- "The best thing you can do for your patients with chronic diseases is to let them run with the ball ... effective chronic illness care requires two things. First, it requires a team with the patient at the center. Second, it requires active, involved participants – especially an active, involved patient. This model of care can be described using various terms – empowerment, informed choice, patient centered – but they all have the same underlying concept: The patient is at the center and is actively involved in his or her own health care" (Funnell 2000, 47).

This is exciting, provocative, and encouraging. In the form of personal health records, there is a rare opportunity to test a broad variety of hypotheses about the use of electronic health tools controlled in part by patients. Personal health records:

> encompass a wide variety of applications that enable people to collect, view, manage, or share copies of their health information or transactions electronically. Although there are many variants, PHRs are based on the fundamental concept of facilitating an individual's access to and creation of personal health information in a usable computer application that the individual (or a designee) controls. We do not envision PHRs as a substitute for the professional and legal obligation for recordkeeping by health care professionals and entities. However, they do portend a beneficial trend toward greater engagement of consumers in their own health and health care. (Markle Foundation 2006, 2)

With personal health records, patients can view their "official" records (or copies or versions of them) and provide information that might be appropriate for a physician or nurse to include in an electronic health record; and patients and clinicians can communicate swiftly and directly. Most electronic health record manufacturers include a personal health record as a feature or adjunct to the electronic record. As with the electronic records themselves, this means that many personal health records in use are provided on an as-is basis and cannot be customized. Moreover, like the larger electronic record system, personal health records are not usually interoperable; that is, a personal health record tethered to a particular hospital's electronic patient record is not likely to be accessible by anyone who lacks privileges at that hospital.

At any rate, these new tools are seen to hold great promise for providing patients, especially those with chronic maladies, with a larger role in their own care, and for supporting health care research and the education of clinicians and patients (Phelps et al. 2014; Mandl and Kohane 2008; Tang et al. 2006; for a more cautionary note, see de Lusignan et al. 2014; and regarding the intersection of social networking and personal genetic testing, see Esposito and Goodman 2009); patients themselves believe these tools could improve their health (Markle Foundation 2008). This is adequate to commend another ethical obligation, a modification to EO 3:

> *Enable easy use of personal health records and conduct more research on their usability, design features, efficacy, and effectiveness.* (EO 3.1)

The point about research cannot be overstated. We have a lot to learn. Preliminary research is fertile (Brennan et al. 2010; Johnson 2010), and early efforts to identify ethical issues are suggestive. They also provide a good introduction to the idea that applied ethics is rarely useful in isolation. In bioethics, or the study of ethical issues arising in health practice, policy, and research, they are often closely related to legal and social issues. This recognition was formalized in 1990 when the US Human Genome Project included an Ethical, Legal and Social Implications (ELSI) Research Program as a core component of its mission (cf. McEwen et al. 2014). (That there is yet no ELSI program in biomedical informatics is an unhappy mystery.) Ethical, legal, and social issues can be particularly difficult to disentangle in studies of health information technology and, relatedly, information and communication technology. ("ICT" studies are better known in Europe than in the United States, and apply to several fields of practice and inquiry beyond the health sciences.) Here is one way to map the personal health record's ELSI space:

- Privacy and confidentiality
  - granular control over PHR disclosure
  - ubiquitous monitoring to generate PHR data
  - cohort effects and vulnerable populations using PHRs
  - social networking reliance of PHRs
  - legal uncertainty regarding nontraditional actors

- Data security
  - challenges of PHR data protection in distributed environments

- Decision support
  - when provided to patients without clinical intermediaries and in extraclinical settings

- Legal-regulatory environment
  - multiple federal requirements and state requirements for PHR-based data and new environments, all of which are evolving, leaving us with few if any standards (adapted with modifications from Cushman et al. 2010, S52).

It was also determined that there are many ethical duties to go around, and it is reasonable to require that patients take some responsibility for the management of their information – at least once they become partners in controlling it. To be sure, these issues are specific, some perhaps unique, to personal health records. Writ larger, many other issues related to privacy, decision support, governance and regulation, and so on will also apply; these and other issues are taken up in subsequent chapters. One of the interesting yet not surprising findings of this initial ELSI survey was that the willingness to share information using a personal health record seemed to correlate with age; that is, younger people were more willing to make their health information available via the Web and perhaps using a mobile device, apparently without clear security measures (cf. Carrión et al. 2012). Although there are several possible explanations for this, it does augur a dynamic future course – which itself is a kind of tacit index of the need for more and ongoing research.

Innovation – and good innovation

We are rarely so aflutter with or excited by change as by change in information technology. No one will queue overnight to acquire the latest model of a car or bicycle, buy the newest organic apple, or procure the hottest West End or Broadway ticket. Announce the availability of the latest cellphone or personal digital assistant, however, and we cannot but help wonder at our compatriots' spare time to do just that (others will queue for lottery tickets, or for jobs). Contrarily, the electronic health record has in important respects reached a kind of stasis: After committing hundreds of millions of dollars, Euros, pesos, or pounds to a new system, no hospital or health care system will be quick to change, and, in any case, innovation is generally proprietary and difficult to compare between and among vendors (see Chapter 6). Lovers of unfettered markets should be encouraged to wonder at how difficult it is to choose among competing electronic health record systems based on price and quality – criteria which we might have hoped would govern such purchases, especially when made at least in part with tax money.

Although biomedical research using electronic health records is evolving quickly (see Chapter 8), rigorous studies comparing them are, apparently, nonexistent. For all we know, the best available open-source system can produce results better and elicit user satisfaction greater than anything on the market.

As we have seen so far and will reaffirm throughout this book, there is no alternative to electronic health records; there never was. What remains now is to improve them so they work well; this is, as above, an ethical obligation. Even marginal improvements are welcome, although they should not engender complacency; because we are, basically, concerned with human suffering and death, the stakes are much too high for that. When the resource baseline is low, however, electronic health records can realize significant gains. The reasonable demand in all domains for measurable goals and objectives is sometimes easy to meet.

Consider the use of electronic patient records in low- and middle-income countries. From HIV care (Were et al. 2011; Were et al. 2013) to nutrition (Lim et al. 2009) and respiratory infections (Diero et al. 2006), Bill Tierney and colleagues at Indiana University's Regenstrief Institute have demonstrated that even the simplest electronic record system can be transformational in otherwise under-resourced medical systems (Rotich et al. 2003; this issue is briefly revisited in Chapter 7). This is good, wholesome, and compelling. Moreover, it applies an insight from some of the very earliest work in ethics and biomedical informatics, namely, that there are times when the availability of a useful tool carries with it a duty to use that tool (Miller et al. 1985). Put differently, ethics is too often used to prohibit or censure, but there are many instances in which a new tool compels us to adopt it (Goodman 2011). This theme will be revisited throughout this book.

Some innovations are incremental, some large and bold. What is wanted in biomedical informatics is a suite of conceptual tools to capture our best instincts to ensure that values we generally embrace are also reflected in system design and use. We can therefore add another ethical obligation:

Embed ELSI considerations in the design and implementation of electronic health records and personal health records. (EO 5)

This is an overarching duty, and it recognizes that the tools of applied ethics are of practical use in shaping good practice, building trust, and protecting patients and communities. To restate the obligations identified so far:

Improve electronic health records. (EO 1)

Expand research on electronic health records. (EO 2)

Foster and support patient access to and control of their information. (EO 3)

Enable easy use of personal health records and conduct more research on their usability, design features, efficacy, and effectiveness. (EO 3.1)

Improve usability by addressing and accommodating human factors, social and organizational issues, and system research. (EO 4)

Embed ELSI considerations in the design and implementation of electronic health records and personal health records. (EO 5)

The list is not intended to be dispositive, or exhaustive. There are doubtless others that could be added; and those enumerated here could be refined. Understood correctly, the job of applied ethics is not to lay down rules or to identify and punish those who break them. Rather, it is to guide professionals who, one hopes, have no objection to the incorporation of ethical considerations in their work. As we will see in Chapter 4, attention to ethics in practice is constitutive of what it means to be a professional in the first place.

All subsequent chapters will provide opportunities to add to our list. Students might productively be asked to do that – that is, to identify ethical obligations related to decision support, privacy, professionalism, and so on. The biomedical informatics community has for decades welcomed the attention of bioethics, and, if nothing else is accomplished here, that relationship will be honored and expanded.

Bioethics and health information technology (revisited)

Nearly 20 years ago appeared the first book-length attempt to identify and assess the ethical issues that arise in health information technology (Goodman 1998a). There was nothing in it about the Internet or World Wide Web. Subsequent advances in the use of computers in the practice of nursing and medicine, in hospital operations, and in biomedical research have been so fast, large, and significant as to make clear that ethics should be included in any identification of the fields that bear on health information technology. What was clear two decades ago, moreover, remains apt today: We have apparently contradictory missions in using computers in health care. One is to use new technology according as it improves health care, and the other is to do so wisely, thoughtfully, and even cautiously. But the air of contradiction can be resolved, and was, with the introduction of the idea of "progressive caution." Here is how it was initially framed:

> The future of the health professions is computational ... This suggests nothing quite so ominous as artificial doctors and robo-nurses playing out "what have we wrought?" scenarios in future cyberhospitals. It does suggest that the standard of care for information acquisition, storage, processing, and retrieval is changing rapidly, and health professionals need to move swiftly or be left behind. Because we are talking about health care, the stakes are quite high. The very idea of a standard of care in the context of pain, life, suffering, health,

and death points directly to a vast ensemble of *ethical* issues. Failing to adhere to publicly defensible standards is to risk or do harm, which, without some overriding justification or reason, is unethical. (Goodman 1998b, 1)

And here is how the idea was summarized:

[T]the most appropriate course to take is one we may call "progressive caution": Medical informatics is, happily, here to stay, but users and society have extensive responsibilities to ensure that we use our tools appropriately. This might cause us to move more deliberately or slowly than some would like. Ethically speaking, that is just too bad. (ibid., 9)

The health care enterprise has a distinctive ability to create compelling labels, some of which seem on analysis to be redundant or tautologous: "evidence-based medicine," as if we'd want any other kind; "comparative effectiveness research," as if most studies were not trying to find out what works best; "meaningful use," as if we might consider, perhaps for the sake of completeness, meaningless use. Yet the intentions are good and wise and may be credited with trying to identify and begin to get a grip on extraordinarily complex systems and processes. We should intend to make ethics a full partner in all these initiatives, especially, for our purposes here, because they are all information-intensive. Indeed, the evolution of networked learning health care systems linking clinical care, genomics, research, and public health – and the challenges this poses to winning and maintaining public trust – makes it clearer that the job of ethics now includes navigational support by applying Progressive Caution for managing uncertainty in increasingly complex systems.

This book tries to do some of that navigation:

Chapter 2 considers computational decision support, one of the most interesting and challenging issues at the intersection of ethics, information technology, and health care. The chapter mulls and answers the question, "If our goal is an accurate diagnosis and prognosis, then what and how does it matter if these are rendered by humans or homunculi, robots or automata, by computers?"

Privacy and confidentiality are the issues most quickly and frequently identified at that intersection. Chapter 3 provides a philosophical foundation for these values and proceeds to justify this conclusion: Privacy and confidentiality are precious – but not absolute.

Now that health informatics is a professional discipline, with special training, board exams, and so on, it is important to be clear about the foundations, scope, and challenges to professionalism. Chapter 4 examines computer-mediated skill degradation, copying and pasting in electronic health records, issues in the responsible conduct of research, and the problem of reproducibility or corroboration of study results.

Chapter 5 provides a response to concerns about patient safety, including an analysis of standards in health information technology. The large, controversial, and difficult problem of system interoperability is the topic of an extended discussion; interoperability itself is cast as an ethical issue and obligation.

Building on prior mention of the role of responsibility and accountability, Chapter 6 examines the role of the electronic health record industry, proposes a number of duties for vendors, and advocates a "patient-centered health information technology industry."

The Internet and World Wide Web, along with mobile health applications, personal care robots, and telehealth, have changed and will continue to change the way people access health care and health care information. This elicits a suite of important ethical issues, discussed in Chapter 7.

From laboratories to learning health systems, the growth of knowledge is driven by research. Chapter 8 offers a sustained review and analysis of ethical issues raised by the use of computers to collect, store, and analyze data and information about humans, along the way emphasizing public health, undermining the concept of "secondary use," contemplating the place for "citizen science," and extolling the role of "trusted governance" in a world in which, it seems, nearly everything generates data.

Two appendices – codes of ethics from major professional organizations – are included as a resource for students.

Regarding students: Ethics, like writing computer code or rendering a nursing or medical diagnosis, is sometimes easy and sometimes not. In either case, however, one might get it wrong. That is, software engineering and the practice of nursing or medicine are guided and governed by criteria. So is ethics. The criteria for making a good argument are rather well established, and if one does not hew to them, one is more likely than not to get the wrong answer. But the temptation to believe that, because it is not empirical or evidence based, ethics is somehow loosey-goosey or not rigorous is a temptation to be resisted. This is worth mentioning because of the frequency of the view, often embraced by students, that "there is no right ethical answer," and the stance, also sadly common, that disagreement constitutes disrespect. Both are wrongheaded, and connected. Ethics thrives on arguments, and counterarguments, on debate. But that is the process, not the goal. The goal is to arrive at the best-possible answer; reasoned disagreement can help us get there. No one upon witnessing two physicians debating a diagnosis at morning report or grand rounds infers from the disagreement that both are right. No one would say, "Well, look at those physicians disagreeing – it looks like anything goes in medicine." What we do say is that more data, more information, or more knowledge is needed to get the correct answer. Although ethics does not use data or information the same way as nursing or medicine, its conclusions are not any less right for that.

Notes

1. This papyrus is missing many pieces, and philologists have made a number of inferences, some of them discordant. Nevertheless, looking through the cases – translations are available at www.reshafim.org.il/ad/egypt/timelines/topics/kahunpapyrus.htm – is rewarding in several ways. For instance, the first case in the world's oldest medical text quite literally addresses pains in the neck, or cervicalgia (for which, in treatment, "thou shalt make her eat the liver of an ass, raw"). Other cases address pain in teeth, feet, ears, vulva, legs, and pelvis, making this artifact also the first to address pain management.

   Lawyers, risk managers, and humorists interested in disclaimers for information technology systems will appreciate the following, by the Web site's creator, André Dollinger: "N.B. Ancient medical texts are easily mistranslated and misinterpreted. WARNING: Do NOT attempt to diagnose or treat ailments in the light of these texts! ... So you think that such a warning is ridiculous? I agree. But then there are people out there who call phone numbers of characters in TV shows in order to tell them what they think of them." For a potentially more advantageous "caution on reading the Ancient Egyptian writings on health," see the University College London resource at www.digitalegypt.ucl.ac.uk/med/healingdraft.htm.

2. He continues: "To pursue a treatment that could not succeed not only harmed the patient but diminished the standing of the practitioner and the reputation of medicine itself. This viewpoint, which has an uncanny bearing on modern medical practice where much anguish often attends decisions to withdraw or withhold therapy, is stated eloquently in the Hippocratic essay 'The Art'"[note omitted]:

   I will define what I conceive medicine to be. In general terms, it is to do away with the sufferings of the sick, to lessen the violence of their diseases, and to refuse to treat those who are overmastered by their diseases, realizing that in such cases medicine is powerless ... For if a man demand from an art a power over what does not belong to the art, or from nature a power over what does not belong to nature, his ignorance is more allied to madness than to lack of knowledge. For in cases where we have the mastery through the means afforded by a natural constitution or by an art, there we may be craftsmen, but nowhere else.

3. See, for instance, The National Center for Biomedical Ontology (www.bioontology.org/), Rubin et al. (2006), and Yu (2006).

4. Reiser (1991, 905) says of Louis that "Only after repeating his investigation could he bring himself to reveal his findings, which were based on a form of analysis that was as far-reaching as the study's conclusion." This emphasis on reproducibility of results foreshadows an issue that has blossomed in importance as bench scientists and clinical trialists have found reproducibility to be far more elusive in contemporary science than good practice would require or even suggest (Collins and Tabak 2014).

5. Louis did not compare patients who were bled to those who were not; instead, he compared those who came to the hospital early in the course of their disease and were therefore bled early to those who came late and were bled late. "More of the patients who were bled early died. This comparison between two noncomparable prognostic groups would be completely unacceptable today. Also, the tables in the original text contain some disturbing arithmetic mistakes" (Vandenbroucke 1998, 2001; cf. Goodman 2003). Nevertheless, he found in these cohorts that "the amount, timing, or frequency of the bleeding had no influence on the outcome and that any apparent effect could be attributed to either a wrong diagnosis or to the use of bloodletting in a patient whose disease had nearly run its course" (Reiser 1991, 905).

6. This was first suggested to me a decade ago by a colleague, Bob Schwartz, chair of the University of Miami Miller School of Medicine's Department of Family Medicine and Community Health.

7. The eight:

    1. **Enhance physicians' ability to provide high-quality patient care.** Poor EHR design gets in the way of face-to-face interaction with patients because physicians are forced to spend more time documenting required information of questionable value. Features such as pop-up reminders, cumbersome menus, and poor user interfaces can make EHRs far more time consuming than paper charts ... Instead, EHRs should be designed to enable physician-patient engagement. Technology should fit seamlessly into the practice and be based on work flow needs.

    2. **Support team-based care.** Current technology often requires physicians to enter data or perform tasks that other team members should be empowered to complete. EHR systems instead should be designed to maximize each person's productivity in accordance with state licensure laws and allow physicians to delegate tasks as appropriate.

    3. **Promote care coordination.** Transitioning patient care can be a challenge without full EHR interoperability and robust tracking. EHR systems need to automatically track referrals, consultations, orders and labs so physicians easily can follow the patient's progression throughout their care.

    4. **Offer product modularity and configurability.** Few EHR systems are built to accommodate physicians' practice patterns and work flows, which vary depending on size, specialty and setting. Making EHR systems more modular would allow physicians to configure their health IT environment to best suit their work flows and patient populations. Allowing vendors to focus on specialized applications also would produce the tailored technology physicians need.

    5. **Reduce cognitive work load.** Although physicians spend significant time navigating their EHR systems, many physicians say that the quality of the clinical narrative in paper charts is more succinct and reflective of the pertinent clinical information. A lack of context and overly structured data capture requirements, meanwhile, can make interpretation difficult.

        EHRs need to support medical decision-making with concise, context-sensitive real-time data. To achieve this, IT developers may need to create sophisticated tools for reporting, analyzing data and supporting decisions. These tools should be customized for each practice environment.

    6. **Promote interoperability and data exchange.** Data "lock in" is a common problem. EHR systems should facilitate connected health care across care settings and enable both exporting data and properly incorporating data from other systems. The end result should be a coherent longitudinal patient record that is built from various sources and can be accessed in real time.

7. **Facilitate digital patient engagement.** Most EHR systems are not designed to support digital patient engagement. But incorporating increased interoperability between EHR systems and patients' mobile technologies and telehealth technologies would be an asset for promoting health and wellness and managing chronic illnesses.

8. **Expedite user input into product design and post-implementation feedback.** The meaningful use program requires physicians to use certified EHR technology, but many of these products have performed poorly in real-world practice settings. EHR systems should give users an automated option to provide context-sensitive feedback that is used to improve system performance and safety.

8. From a social networking site for HP Nano: www.facebook.com/HPNnano/posts/422122111199195. Cf. the Robert Wood Johnson Foundation's Project HealthDesign: www.projecthealthdesign.org/. Some of the material here on personal health records was shaped by a 2006–2008 Robert Wood Johnson Foundation grant to the University of Miami and this author. See www.projecthealthdesign.org/artifacts/artifacts-elsi.

Ancient professions and intelligent machines
The ethical challenge of computational decision support

This chapter addresses what is arguably the most interesting and difficult issue that arises at the intersection of ethics, computing, and the health professions: when, by whom, under what circumstances, and with what training should a human use a computer to make or support a medical diagnosis or prognosis? What does medicine consist in if computers render more accurate diagnoses and prognoses than humans? When does it become blameworthy not to use a medical decision support system or prognostic scoring system if evidence suggests improved outcomes? For now, there is inadequate warrant to believe that computers can consistently outperform humans. This means that if we want an exception to the too-oft-repeated scenario in which technology outstrips ethics, then marshaling the tools of applied ethics now will prepare us for the era of thinking machines that do some things better than humans.

Humans, machines, and clinical decision making

An accurate diagnosis is a beautiful thing. Mommies and daddies make them all the time, as do nurses, psychologists, and physicians. Some practitioners are self-effacing after an accurate but difficult diagnosis, in the way medical-school educators try to guide and shape their students, and others are self-impressed, arrogant hydrocodone addicts, in the way television tries to undo all that. Do we prefer smart and edgy or warm and fuzzy for our diagnoses? Cold, hard, and accurate, or warm, soft, and human? Perhaps a hybrid would be best: A human who always figured it out, always got the right answer; or a robot that did the same, while holding a hand or brushing a tear ...

The great Paracelsus, a mad, syphilitic sixteenth-century physician, mercury addict, and alchemist, who introduced chemistry to medicine and founded occupational medicine, was on an interesting tack when he channeled the automata of antiquity in claiming to create, through ectogenesis, a homunculus using human blood and sperm, and horse manure.[1] His was the first in a line of homunculi, thought by some to be able to predict the future, and said to have inspired aspects of Goethe's *Faust*. Doubtless the physician Paracelsus would want his creation to have a go at medicine. Now, a homunculus physician would be very creepy indeed, though we should imagine for a moment one which (who?) always got the diagnosis and prognosis right. Would that be more tolerable than a mechanical, metal robot because of the blood and sperm? Or do we care much at all for its composition, as long as it is able to get it right? Nice and wrong versus creepy and right.

Put differently, if our goal is an accurate diagnosis and prognosis, then what and how does it matter if these are rendered by humans or homunculi, robots or automata, by computers?

Assigning the property "intelligence" to a machine, as in the title of this book, is unintentionally provocative. It implies that a clinical decision support system – a computer, database(s), and software that renders diagnoses and differential diagnoses – may be said to be "intelligent" in the same way, more or less, as humans or other animals possess an ability to learn, to use one language or another, to follow or obey rules of inference or logic, and even perhaps to have understanding. It might be best to regard "intelligence" in this context as a metaphor. Any unease at the idea of a successful computational diagnostician was present before we called it "intelligent." Even a successful medical Turing test, in which, say, patients could not tell whether they were being diagnosed by a human or a machine, would tell us little about the practice of medicine, there being more to such practice than quiz-show-like guessing by the inexpert. What matters here, and is the project for this chapter, is an account of appropriate uses and users of diagnostic and prognostic machines. It is not a technical question, or a narrow one. It is about nothing less than what it means to practice medicine or nursing and, whether there is something, or anything, essentially or necessarily human about such practice. Ethical issues raised by computational diagnosis are at least as interesting as any in the world of biomedical informatics, given the very idea that a machine, intelligent or otherwise, might be able to perform a function that for millennia has been something only humans do, could do, or do well. Consider these questions (cf. Goodman 2014; and, more grandly, Moor 1979):

- Can intelligent machines practice medicine or nursing?
- Is there anything exclusively or essentially human about the practice of medicine or nursing?
- What does clinical practice consist in besides rendering diagnoses and prognoses? Whatever that turns out to be, could machines do it, too?
- When, if ever, is it permissible to use an intelligent machine in the practice of medicine or nursing?
- Is it possible that one day it will be obligatory to use an intelligent machine in the practice of medicine? Will that be a good thing?

Deciding whether and when to use a new tool can be one of the most difficult challenges in clinical practice. To adopt an instrument, a drug, or device without understanding how it works can be a source of serious mischief in patient care. But failure to use a tool that has been shown to improve patient care does a different kind of mischief: medicine, nursing, and the other health professions progress in part because practitioners are able, at least eventually, to recognize when standards are changing, and when failure to change with them can mean inferior care for patients.

The questions of what is inferior or superior and what ought to be the standard are likewise very difficult and very interesting. The notion of a standard of care, whose rich complexities we bury beneath a simple and apparently straightforward phrase, has important consequences in ethics and law. A clinician who is too far behind the times may be faulted for failing to use tools that have been shown to improve patient care. But a clinician who is too far ahead of the times may also be faulted for not providing the standard of care (although this usually only occurs if something goes wrong). Sometimes, progress consists in successfully providing care that is not standard, but which increases or moves the standard forward. There can even be an imperative to do something that makes sense even if it is not the standard.[2]

Diagnosis

A diagnosis is a kind of hypothesis, inferred to be accurate based on signs and symptoms and more-or-less well-justified beliefs about the accuracy of previous uses of the (name of the) diagnosis. One can make a diagnosis that leads to a successful treatment, but be wrong about the reason: If Hippocrates or Paracelsus, say, were to have diagnosed a patient with an imbalance of bodily humors such that blood was out of equilibrium with phlegm, black bile, and green bile, and then ordered a bloodletting, then every time a patient felt better would constitute a reason to suppose the diagnosis was correct; in fact, bloodletting can be successful in the management of a patient with hemochromatosis or porphyria cutanea tarda, though Hippocrates and Paracelsus could not have known that it was hemochromatosis or porphyria cutanea tarda they were successfully treating. The humoral theory is false, but could appear to be confirmed. That appearance of confirmation demonstrates how a diagnosis can seem to identify or label a causal chain, but not in fact do so.[3]

The diagnosis can have economic or political importance. Nowadays, we assign codes to diagnoses, generally to improve public health and support epidemiology and, in some jurisdictions, to undergird the process of billing for medical services. The International Statistical Classification of Diseases, maintained by the World Health Organization,[4] is a complex and sweeping set of alphanumeric identifiers. (The ICD-10 code for hemochromatosis is E83.119; this, in turn, is located under the diagnosis-related group 642 for "inborn and other disorders of metabolism.") The ICD system is a vast, computable constellation of identifiers, which, with SNOMED, maintained by the International Health Terminology Standards Development Organisation,[5] are the world's largest-ever classifications of diseases and health care terminology. Created in the tradition of Sauvages, Linnaeus, and Graunt, the ICD system is imperfect and so illustrates nicely that the task of diagnosis is presently not and, might never be, perfect or precise:

> While three centuries have contributed something to the scientific accuracy of disease classification, there are many who doubt the usefulness of attempts to compile statistics of disease, or even causes of death, because of the difficulties of classification. To these, one can quote Major Greenwood: "The scientific purist, who will wait for medical statistics until they are nosologically exact, is no wiser than Horace's rustic waiting for the river to flow away."
> (World Health Organization 2010, 163; citing Greenwood 1948; cf. Engelhardt 1985)

This challenge, or difficulty, will be put to use in arriving at the conclusion of this chapter.

An accurate diagnosis, even if premised on faulty theory, could be of great economic, public relations, and political use. Roger French, in a discomfiting analysis of the social and economic evolution of medical practice, sees diagnosis as a lever for the social status of ancient physicians:

> The converse of ethics seen in this light is the Greek doctor's need to recognise hopeless cases, so that he could avoid them. This looks timelessly unethical to us, but it meant that the doctor could avoid being linked to failure, that is, death. Greek prognosis was not only a matter of predicting an outcome; it also involved diagnosis in the sense of persuading the patient that the doctor knew about the condition itself. In describing the symptoms to the patient, perhaps symptoms that the patient had forgotten to mention, the doctor could make a display of his technical knowledge that would impress the patient and family. This

knowledge was valuable. Indeed, it was a stock-in-trade that the doctor used two ways: to treat his patients and to maintain the reputation of the group to which he belonged. Some groups were aware of this to the extent of keeping their medical knowledge secret ...

(French 2003, 16; notes omitted).

(It is tempting but would be mean-spirited to suggest that something similar is occurring with electronic health record vendors refusing to make public the screenshots and other details of their programs; see below.) As ever, efforts to find or make a diagnosis might mean that someone will get paid.

Diagnosis has been a method of solving problems (Simon 1985), the result or process of following any number of logics (Sadegh-Zadeh 2012), and the synthesis of evidence applied to individual patients (Goodman 2003). It carries the ineffable power of a name as applied to one of the greatest of human concerns – a lack or absence of well-being. It confers authority, signals competence if not expertise, offers a sense of command, at least if it is true that to name something is to claim some measure of control over it. This is especially valuable in the absence of any treatment, as has been the case for most maladies for most of the history of civilization. In modern clinical science, there are numerous treatments, and some or many actually work. A diagnosis is a pointer to a treatment, a path to a prognosis, and a cairn on the road to a cure.

Computational decision support

Consider a hypothetical computer system that consistently, reliably, and accurately delivers diagnoses and treatment plans. At the point of care, at the bedside of the sleeping patient, a clinician consults her tablet or personal digital assistant. The Certified Clinical Advanced Program for Official Long-term Laboratory Operations (CC-Apollo) system has full and fast access to the patient's electronic health record and an app that runs the EHR data through a diagnostic engine and a library of practice guidelines. The device provides a diagnosis and several differential diagnoses, each with a likelihood or probability of being correct, along with a list of tests one might do to rule out each of them, in an easy-to-read and intuitive user interface. The diagnosis is correct, as it always is. Several treatments are recommended and ranked, including one for a specially titrated drug based on genomic information in the electronic health record. In addition to clinical and physiological data and information, the device and app process social information, including material about the patient's family, occupation, and lifestyle. A comprehensive interview on admission had elicited facts about patient values on such topics as death and dying, disability, and willingness to have anonymized data and information made available for analysis under a protocol approved by the research ethics committee or institutional review board.

The clinician taps "OK" and the diagnosis is entered into the electronic health record with the clinician's name and ID, the version and build of the diagnostic expert system, and time stamped. The drug is ordered and delivered and administered the next day. The patient is discharged in a week and lives another 30 months, dying peacefully and at home just two weeks after the birth of his first grandchild, whom he was able to hold for several minutes (i.e., until his daughter decided that was quite enough). An automatic "service history for information technology" review found that this patient lived 10–12 months longer and with higher functional status than the 99 other patients in the province with the same diagnosis during the preceding year – longer and better than the 70 others whose institutions did not use CC-Apollo and the 29 whose institutions did use the system but where the interns and residents chose to override the primary diagnosis and ordered batteries of tests to rule out all the differentials. The system had warned that such tests can increase morbidity and mortality and lengthen hospital stay, with correlate deconditioning.

There is of course no "CC-Apollo" system,[6] but if there were, would you use it for your patients or insist that your doctor or nurse did? Better, imagine one of your own. Make it flawless and easy to use. Make it cheap, or free. The key component of this thought experiment is that it involves a decision support system that renders accurate diagnoses and effective treatment plans. Patients for whom it is used will fare better than those who are managed and treated by humans with no decision support tool. The goal or point here is to focus narrowly on the question whether a particular tool improves patient care. In all other areas of practice, if a procedure, approach, drug, device, or any other tool were to be accompanied by clear evidence that it worked better than the alternatives, it would be irrational, even negligent, not to use it, and perhaps absurd not to require its use.

So, does this perfect decision support system *improve patient care*?

Our CC-Apollo system user never examines, never speaks to, and never touches her patient. Is there a "doctor–patient relationship"? If the patient awoke just then, he would not recognize her. If the shared goal here is not suffering, not losing function or ability, and/or not being dead, what difference does it make who or what renders the diagnosis? What difference does it make if there is no relationship to enjoy and celebrate? What difference does it make if there is less on-the-job satisfaction for the clinical team?

Surely, to press this point, it would be the height of hubris to allow our love of the health professions and our pride in their successes to be used to justify shunning a tool if it improved patient care, to allow ourselves to be so beguiled by our own history and satisfaction that we put our gratification ahead of the well-being of patients. Indeed it would. *However* – and here we shift course – we remain far from any system that even resembles CC-Apollo; there is not now and will not be for the foreseeable future anything so good as to abjure the role of competent humans; and we are more likely to be beguiled by our systems than by our professional pride. It is best now to explore this new course. The exploration must be undertaken against an extraordinary backdrop: There are hundreds of decision support and prognostic scoring systems, sometimes called "clinical calculators," most apparently freely available on the Web. It would be interesting to know how many clinicians are aware of them and use any of them. They range from London's King's College Hospital Criteria for liver failure to Washington's National Institute of Child Health and Human Development's "Extremely Preterm Birth Outcome Calculator" and from oncology to psychiatry.[7]

Alarms, electronic order entry, and user interfaces

In the first sustained treatment of ethical issues in biomedical informatics, some three decades ago, by a physician, philosopher, and a lawyer, it was noted that decision support systems and other computational tools were getting better but far from perfect, but that if a tool could be seen or demonstrated to improve care, then it ought to be used (Miller et al. 1985).[8] This struck a balance between boosters and Luddites and has shaped or informed the ethical analysis of computational decision support ever since. The question whether and when to adopt a new tool is rarely answered dramatically. Rather, change is slow and progress is accretive. Decision support functionality of various rudimentary kinds is already a feature in all commercial electronic health record systems and therefore a part of quotidian hospital care, at least. Here is a testable hypothesis: A nontrivial number of well-educated, non-clinically trained, and perhaps overconfident family members of hospitalized patients have, after a few days of listening to alarms sound from pulse, oxygen saturation, and breathing monitors, pressed the "silence" button on the monitor. Doubtless inspired by the annoying sound (where the property of being annoying is itself an essential feature), such family members somehow acquire the belief that silencing the alarm will not harm the patient or cause or allow the patient to be harmed, *and they are right*. Put differently: If laypeople could be comfortable silencing an alarm, what does this entail for professionals?

Alarms, alerts, and reminders are comparatively easy to write code for, and to ignore. While the ability of reminder systems to improve care has long been documented, the utility of alarms has been underwhelming, in large part because of "alarm fatigue" and false alarms.[9] How could such a good and potentially life-saving idea not work as intended? There are several possible reasons: unacceptable false positive and/or false negative rates, inapt user interfaces, discordance with established workflow, and insufficient or inadequate education. Seen as hypotheses, all are equally plausible (see, e.g., McCoy et al. 2012; Nanji et al. 2014; van der Sijs et al. 2006). Overarchingly, the best explanation for the failure of most health information technology applications is probably "all of the above" – but with a twist: many failures could be prevented if the system or tool had first been adequately tested, vetted or evaluated in the context of actual use and before it was fully put in place. Surely one would want to test-drive a car on the streets of the city before driving it home (let alone before committing to a fleet).

The idea of system evaluation as an ethical issue or requirement was first articulated in 1998:

> Medical computing is not merely about medicine or computing. It is about the introduction of new tools into environments with established social norms and practices. The effects of computing systems in health care are subject to analysis not only of accuracy and performance but of acceptance by users, of consequences for social and professional interaction, and of the context of use. We suggest that system evaluation can illuminate social and ethical issues in medical computing, and in so doing improve patient care. That being the case, there is an ethical imperative for such evaluation.   (Anderson and Aydin 1998, 57)

It is sad, rare, and, somehow, not surprising that such good advice could be so frequently and so thoroughly ignored. The suggested evaluation regimen is simple to articulate and intuitively straightforward. The gist of what is recommended has been distilled to ten questions (Anderson and Aydin 1994):

1. Does the system work as designed?
2. Is it used as anticipated?
3. Does it produce the desired results?
4. Does it work better than the procedures it replaced?
5. Is it cost effective?
6. How well have individuals been trained to use it?
7. What are the anticipated long-term effects on how organizational units interact?
8. What are the long-term effects on the delivery of medical care?
9. Will the system have an impact on control in the organization?
10. To what extent do effects depend on practice setting?

Any objections? Of course not. Consider a computerized physician order entry system, or CPOE.[10] Depending on whom one asks, CPOE systems reduce error (Radley et al. 2013) or can foster error (Leviss 2013); probably both, depending on context and other factors (Lainer et al. 2013). What seems to be the case is that both the failure to improve prescribing and the active frustration of successful order entry are caused in part by poorly designed user interfaces – a problem addressed or at least touched on by perhaps half of the ten questions just enumerated. Were CPOE systems evaluated in the context of actual use, they would be easier to use, debug, and improve. Were their embedded alerts and reminders assessed by the professionals who would be depending on them, these systems would better be able to improve the quality of care.

Now, the issue of user interfaces has special salience in the world of decision support. If anything about the representation of information or the depiction of clinical options is unclear or confusing, the interface can at the least waste time and, at worst, endanger patients. This suggests an exciting opportunity for any number of research projects to analyze and compare CPOE and other applications (for decision support or otherwise), to measure how different forms of information representation affect the quality of care and clinical outcomes, and to embed patient safety as a core component of the responsible use of health information technology.

It is a pity that none of this is possible.

As it develops, the manufacturers of electronic health records, order-entry systems, and their accoutrements regard screenshots of their user interfaces as a kind of intellectual property to be protected, and, therefore, systematically restrict public sharing or disclosure of these images. This is apparently true even if the sharing and disclosure are for research, quality improvement, and so on. In one case, a 2014 report to the US Food and Drug Administration "on CPOE interfaces that are associated with medication error risks and often with actual errors" by a consortium of universities was withheld from public access to prevent disclosure of screenshots.[11] This is as mysterious as it is troubling. It is mysterious because (i) most user interfaces are not very good, so it is hard to believe there is much risk of them being stolen or emulated; (ii) legitimate investigators, scholars, and others have long been and regularly are entrusted with sensitive intellectual property and corporate data – as, for instance, on institutional review boards or research ethics committees; and (iii) the usual way to protect an image is by registering a copyright, not hiding the image. It is troubling because it (i) impedes research and quality improvement, (ii) therefore reduces patient safety, and (iii) hence violates uncontroversial business values and standards for transparency and account-ability (see Chapter 6).

If the full potential of alarms, alerts, reminders, and order-entry systems is to be realized, they must be treated the same as any other clinical tool. (See Gotz et al. 2014 for an interesting use of visual analysis itself.) They must, that is, be analyzed and studied by competent investigators in public forums. We have seen in less than a decade a transformation of drug and device research such that clinical trials now increasingly must be registered in advance, results must be publicly available even if not published after peer review, and even published results must include pointers to online data sets. If drug and device industry data, the cradle of most of the medical intellectual property in the history of civilization, can thus be made public, then surely the makers of electronic health records can share their data and its representations, including pictures of user interfaces, without too much financial damage and especially given that many of these systems were paid for and are sustained with tax money. Indeed, if we really cared about patient safety, such sharing would be easy, encouraged, and, indeed, required by civil society.

Education as an ethical imperative

The importance of training, if not education, has been hinted at in several places here so far. It would be truly remarkable if the electronic and computational transformation of health care could be achieved by clinicians who shared secret notes (a kind of professional samizdat), read a few articles, or got the inside scoop on CPOE from characters of questionable reputation, on the streets. That is, effective and responsible use of all tools, and including those that process information, requires a solid understanding of the tools' purposes, functions, and mechanisms. It especially requires attention to the relationship between the human and the tool.

Perhaps the most widespread of all nontrivial decision support tools is the drug dosing and interaction alert. Here is a key step in the Meaningful Use attestation process under the US Centers for Medicare and Medicaid Services:

> Certified EHRs with the drug interaction checks enabled gives real-time information on possible interactions at the time of ordering, minimizing the potential for adverse events or pharmacy call-backs. With many patients taking nutritional supplements, having medications provided from multiple providers, or allergies to certain medications – having a drug interaction check provides better clinical decisions by displaying alerts on drug-allergy, drug-frequency, drug-drug, drug-renal function, drug-laboratory, and drug-age which can improve the safety and effectiveness of medication.[12]

This in turn requires that systems "Enable the severity level of interventions provided for drug-drug interaction checks to be adjusted [and …] Limit the ability to adjust severity levels to an identified set of users or available as a system administrative function." This raises the question of appropriate severity levels and calls for determination of circumstances in which prescriptions may be overridden and when they may not be, when and how either setting may be questioned or appealed, the acceptable grounds for such a question or appeal, and so on. If overrides are a measure of appropriate or valid settings, then high override rates suggest that the process is disappointing (Bryant et al. 2014; more optimistically, see Phansalkar et al. 2014). Perhaps a maiden-voyage issue, these kinds of challenges nevertheless point more broadly to the need for CPOE users to have at least some understanding of how the settings and limits are arrived at. In some cases, it might be a mistake to override the system (the user was unaware of a recent update to an allergy list [though this points to an additional and different problem]), and in another instance it might be a mistake not to override the system (imagine limits on opioid analgesia use set by someone or some process ignorant of the needs of palliative care).

Making CPOE and other decision support users partners in establishing the functionality of the tools they use is good common sense – and the way to begin that partnership is through education in system structure and design, and emphatically not merely in a canned how-to-use-the-system online tutorial. We should not resist the fantasy of a suite of smart and engaging curricula which themselves are evaluated for pedagogic quality and effectiveness. (To be sure, such curricula would need to make liberal use of system screenshots.) Any sort of mere how-to training that explicitly or tacitly signals learners to "pay no attention to that man behind the curtain," that is, to disregard the system's empirical or scientific underpinnings, would be unacceptable in any other area of clinical practice – just imagine telling a physician that a particular drug is indicated for a specific malady, but that she need not be bothered by the drug's mechanism of action. Meaningful use will be especially meaningful when the equivalent of magic, blind faith, or willful ignorance is impermissible as part of a causal explanation.

This need for high-quality educational resources will increase, perhaps dramatically, as genomic data acquire greater importance in electronic health records, and computerized physician order entry will be expected to navigate and guide users through ever-finer-grained pharmacogenomic decision paths (see, e.g., Devine et al. 2014; Goldspiel et al. 2014; and Overby et al. 2012; for assessments from the steadily growing legal literature, see, e.g., Hoffman and Podgurski 2012; and Ridgely and Greenberg 2012). The stakes for patients will be higher than ever, and the need for bona fide insight into the workings of drug-interaction engines will trump any argument suggesting that less is better, that the details are inessential, or that intellectual property is more precious or more deserving of protection than patient safety.[13]

Diagnostic systems

As made clear at the outset of this chapter, the fullest or largest expression of our challenge is this: If computers can consistently make more accurate diagnoses than humans, then what does this mean for the practice of medicine or nursing, and by what lights should we navigate in these new waters? When is it accurate to say the standard of care has changed – or should change? Has it changed yet?

Surely not. Computerized decision support systems cannot yet do all of the dramatic things so far mentioned – especially surpass humans at diagnostic acumen, despite decades of optimism (cf. Pauker and Kassirer 1981). This should not be too great a source of comfort. Computers and programs are consistently and quickly improving, and we ought not wait until they best humans to see how the tools of applied ethics can provide guidance when the day comes when not using a computer to (help) render a diagnosis will be considered foolish. Here is how the problem was introduced elsewhere:

> Based on the uncertainties that surround any new technology, scientific evidence counsels caution and prudence. As in other clinical areas, evidence and reason determine the appropriate level of caution. For instance, there is considerable evidence that electronic laboratory information systems improve access to clinical data when compared with manual, paper-based test-result distribution methods. To the extent that such systems improve care at an acceptable cost in time and money, there is an obligation to use computers to store and retrieve clinical laboratory results. There is a small but growing body of evidence that existing clinical expert systems can improve patient care in a small number of practice environments at an acceptable cost in time and money ... Nevertheless, such systems cannot yet uniformly improve care in typical, more general practice settings, at least not without careful attention to the full range of managerial as well as technical issues affecting the particular care delivery setting in which they are used.
>
> (Goodman et al. 2014, 330–1; this point is due to Randy Miller; references omitted)

This is important, moreover, true, and is, no doubt, good news for those rooting for humans. What is more, the research on decision support systems leaves something, or much, to be desired, in some cases because of low-quality reporting of randomized controlled trials of such systems (Augestad et al. 2012); also, systems are difficult to compare, and individuals or institutions in the market, for one, have precious little data to support their decision (Dhiman et al. 2015; cf. Berner et al. 1994 for an important early comparison of decision support systems); and, in any case, decision support systems seem, so far, to have little effect on actual practice (Pearson et al. 2009) – with no clear sense that those who used such systems should have changed their practice but did not.

The most thoughtful stance to these issues was articulated a quarter century ago by Randy Miller, a physician, decision support system developer, and leader in the informatics community. The Standard View (herein and hereafter a proper noun) is that the *practice of medicine and nursing* are ineluctably human (Miller 1990; see also Friedman 2009). A weak version of the Standard View is that human cognition and intelligence are for the time being more applicable or suited to the task of diagnosis and therefore better at it than machine intelligence; this is why a human diagnosis should not be overridden or trumped by a computer. There are two ways of reading this: either that a human might on reflection come to agree with an initially conflicting computational diagnosis, in which case the human still has the final word, or that no system should ever require acceptance of a computational diagnosis; that is, any such system's diagnosis must always permit a human override. A strong version of the Standard View deletes the "for the time being" proviso, so that if in the future a perfect inference engine were to be introduced, even it should permit human overrides. It is possible to defer defense of that position to the day when there is such a system. A justification of the position could be offered now, however, by arguing that the practice of medicine or nursing have never been and will never be merely or exclusively about the making of accurate inferences. The rendering of a diagnosis will, except in the simplest of cases, always be probabilistic in one degree or another, and induction alone cannot resolve all uncertainty, incorporate human values, or reveal causal relationships necessary for successful clinical practice. That is, humans overwhelmingly understand humans and the problems caused by their maladies better than intelligent machines (Miller 1990). The same is true for artificial intelligence machines that operate with *abductive* inference protocols, where abduction, or, in philosophical parlance, inference to the best explanation, calls for hypotheses about what facts or states of affairs are most likely to support the truth of a finding or, here, diagnosis.

On both the weak and strong versions of the Standard View, the correct approach is to use computers as tools and not replacements for human judgment. This approach recognizes that humans actually make more diagnostic errors than they should,[14] and any tool found to reduce diagnostic error should be used (van den Berge and Mamede 2013; Berner 2014; Newman-Toker and Pronovost 2009; Wachter 2010). Put differently, computerized decision support can improve care when used appropriately (see Mack et al. 2009). This is an ethical requirement as well as a clinical strategy. Moreover, the Standard View captures basic intuitions about quality, including error avoidance, and the ethical responsibilities of clinicians (Goodman et al. 2014).[15]

Appropriate uses and users of diagnostic and prognostic machines

It is difficult if not impossible to identify duties and responsibilities in an empirical vacuum. That is, once we identify the values to which we must hew, we must also have some warrant for beliefs that any particular action or policy is more or less likely to help us do our duties and meet our responsibilities. As we saw in Chapter 1 and will develop further in Chapters 4 and 6, the values to be brought to bear at the intersection of medicine, nursing, dentistry, and so on, information technology and computer science, and the business professions are plural and diverse. If we value patient safety, reliability, and transparency, say, at that intersection, then we will do well to have some evidence of which actions and policies are most likely to make good on the embrace of those values. Education is a universal donor to the project. This is why it was helpful earlier to identify education itself as a kind of supervalue. There is good reason to believe that education and training[16] improve our abilities to protect patient safety, produce reliable products, and foster transparency. There is therefore no surprise in insisting that use of computerized provider order entry and decision support tools be preceded by a thoughtful education regime.

It follows from this that identifying appropriate *users* of these tools will be made easier by being able to pick out those who have been adequately taught both how to use them as well as the conceptual and scientific basis for their use. (This is another reason to support the idea that learners must have access to information about the structure and display of patient and public-health information. There is no room for "secret codes" and concealed user interfaces in high-quality education and training of health professionals using information technology tools.)

Additionally, an appropriate user will be identified by other traits that improve practice, safety, and so on. This is a more complex undertaking, with economic and even political threads. For instance, while it should be uncontroversial to suggest that appropriately trained and educated nurses and physicians should be able to use decision support tools, it is more difficult to identify patients as appropriate users. This is not to say that patients should somehow be forbidden from using a diagnostic expert system; rather, it is to say that an appropriate policy to address such use must be informed by evidence about whether such use harms patients. There is no such evidence, or evidence to the contrary, regarding the consequences of widespread lay use of decision support tools.

Appropriate *uses* will similarly be identified by data about the consequences of permitting various applications.[17] Here is an unordered list of uses of decision support systems that includes the most appropriate and the most inappropriate:

- Determining reimbursement levels
- Improving diagnostic accuracy
- Providing education
- Identifying patients who will cost too much to treat
- Guiding public health policy
- Withdrawing privileges to practice
- Improving billing accuracy
- Credentialing clinicians
- Identifying patients with maladaptive behaviors
- Increasing billing amounts
- Improving workflow

It could be an interesting pedagogic strategy to ask students to add to the list and then argue for or against each use and perhaps to order or rank the list from appropriate use to inappropriate use, and why. Think of values and of information or evidence as interlocking sieves that can filter actions and policies to identify those actions and policies that should be defended or retained, and those that should be abandoned or disdained.

In addition to the responsibilities of clinicians and institutions, it must be underscored that any assessment of appropriate uses and users presumes a foundation of ongoing evaluation and research into the effectiveness of decision support systems, and that findings here make their way into correlate training and education. Moreover, the content, structure, and currency of the databases that undergird any decision support system must – absolutely must – be continuously monitored and revised as needed. It follows that system users need to be able to communicate with each other and with the systems' builders to improve the systems' functionality and accuracy, as well as the ways recommendations are displayed. Surely this is uncontroversial.

Prognostic scoring systems

As above, the Greek physician's ability to diagnose and prognose conferred a number of benefits on the physician and his group. At the beginning of his *Prognosis* Hippocrates suggests as follows:

> One must know to what extent [diseases] exceed the strength of the body and one must have a thorough acquaintance with their future course. In this way one may become a good physician and justly win high fame. In the case of patients who were going to survive, he would be able to safeguard them the better from complications by having a longer time to take precautions. By realizing and announcing beforehand which patients were going to die, [the physician] would absolve himself from any blame. (Hippocrates 1983, 170)

A more patient-centered approach might perhaps inquire in greater detail about the benefit of an accurate diagnosis to a patient. And this, of course, will vary a great deal from patient to patient. Hippocrates seems to have been somewhat mindful about this, seeing the value in patients having "a longer time to take precautions," which is among the reasons contemporary medical educators underscore the importance of communicating adequate information to dying patients; without knowing the prognosis, a patient cannot either gird for the fight or put his affairs in order before dying.

Throughout history, at least in popular culture, the plaintive query "What are my chances, Doc?" has been answered from the hip, the prognosis being based on experience with previous patients, maybe a literature review, and perhaps either wishful thinking or a pessimistic bent. The question is a demand for an essentially probabilistic prediction, which might be high or low. It could also be said to be unavoidably biased, shaped by personal and therefore idiosyncratic experience, cultural values, and other potential confounders of an ability to predict the future accurately. Suppose, however, that a machine could make the necessary calculations and render an accurate prognosis. Would it be less biased and consequently more accurate? Indeed, unless it were programmed to be biased, or the programming language itself could channel programmers' biases, it would likely not be biased.

The virtue of a reliable prognostic scoring system could be that it gives precisely such unbiased and generally accurate predictions. What matters the most ethically is that some or many of these computerized prognoses are predictions regarding whether a particular patient is going to die during a specific hospitalization.

A justified belief that a patient will die within a limited period of time is a very powerful belief. Even if such a belief is no more certain than any other clinical judgment, it could be argued that failure to incorporate that belief into patient care would be irrational. As earlier, imagine a perfect or near-perfect system, that is, one that nearly always predicted whether a patient would survive hospitalization. Given such accuracy, why not use the prognosis to inform end-of-life care decisions? Indeed, prognostic scoring systems are generally designed for use in intensive or critical care units. If an ICU patient is going to die, why keep him in a unit designed for high-intensity care delivered with the goal of maximizing survival? Indeed, and overarchingly, if one does not have enough information to know how a particular patient will fare, more or less – information about his history, available institutional resources, and how he compares to previous and similar patients – then on what basis is high-quality care to be provided in the first place? We need look back only about 200 years to find one of the first expressions of this concern, by the physician William Farr, a student of Pierre Charles Alexandre Louis (recall his "numerical method" from Chapter 1) and mentor of Florence Nightingale, who correlated cholera mortality and water pollution and, conversely, the reduction in mortality from evolving sanitary measures in England (Stroup and Berkelman 1988, 4):

> The enemy of medical progress is the hypothetical or speculative reasoning of physicians. It is time to tell such persons that these vague speculations … are worth nothing and that they can only advance science by registering facts, employing the microscope, by chemical analysis, weighing and measuring phenomena, determining their relations and by applying the mighty instrument of natural science – arithmetic and mathematics. (Farr 1837)[18]

A variation of this passage is cited by William Knaus, developer of the best-known and apparently most widely used of all prognostic scoring systems, APACHE, for Acute Physiology and Chronic Health Evaluation (Knaus 2002, 37).[19] The introduction of APACHE in 1981 (Knaus et al. 1981) was followed by a series of landmark articles in critical care computing (Knaus et al. 1985, 1986, 1991). Thus:

> Our goal in developing APACHE was also to use mathematics more explicatively to monitor the process and evaluate the outcomes of care. We designed APACHE to occupy a middle ground between the attempts to define illness severity by a single number and those requiring extensive and complex mathematical calculations. We also wanted an approach that could be used universally for most patients, but also be precise enough to have relevance for an individual patient. (Knaus 2002, 38)

Prognostic scoring systems are used to analyze critical care outcomes for a number of purposes, including comparing internal outcomes over time, making comparisons between or among institutions, and assessing the status and predicting the survival of individual patients. It was clear both in the early days of APACHE as well as three decades later (e.g., Kramer et al. 2013) that any inferences about the first two uses must take into account a unit's case-mix, lest institutions that customarily treat sicker patients be unfairly judged in comparisons with those whose patients are not as sick.

As discussed above, it is in the use of prognostic scoring systems to predict the risk of death for individual patients that these systems engender the most interesting and difficult ethical issues. If mortality can be more or less accurately predicted, why not use such systems to address, if not partially solve, the ancient problem of clinical futility? Since antiquity, physicians have had at least a rough-and-ready sense whether a patient would survive. It would be empirically strange to contend that in the absence of utter certainty in such prognoses that all available interventions should be aggressively employed to try to prolong the life of the patient. It would be strange because it would be an exception to well-motivated standard practice to make the best decision one can with the best evidence available. This is never a call for infallibility. Rather, it is a demand that clinicians play with the cards they are dealt and make the best decision, or bet, accordingly, or given the best available evidence. Moreover, it would be inapt to reply that, in the case of mortality predictions, the stakes are high enough to warrant overtreatment in an attempt to forestall death, as if there are no bad consequences to giving it a go and failing when failing is most likely. Many bad consequences issue from aggressive and ineffective end-of-life treatment, not least that when the patient does die, he will have done so badly and perhaps painfully because of the additional pain, suffering, and other misadventures that often accompany the attempt. Indeed, many patients are happy and wise to forgo a brief and miserable extension of life in exchange for a peaceful and un-tumultuous death, an option often forfeited with the kind of "therapeutic frenzy" that too often accompanies eleventh-hour lifesaving attempts.

But perhaps too much has been proved. As we saw in the discussion of computational diagnoses, even a flawless system really works only if we reduce clinicians to inference machines and clinical practice to extruding diagnoses and prognoses. Knaus and colleagues saw that "Objective probability estimates will frequently confirm uncertainty regarding the patient's ability to survive. Sometimes confidence intervals will be too large to encourage reliance on the point estimate. These characteristics and the continuous nature of the estimates must be emphasized, lest objective estimates be misunderstood as decision rules, which might restrict rather than enhance clinical reasoning" (Knaus et al. 1991, 392). Moreover, "The value inherent in the system is that medical criteria should form the foundation for decision making and that patients' preferences and values should modify the process" (Knaus 1993, 196). This point is made every generation or so: "But even if we were flawless prognosticators, we would still be left with the larger ethical problem of what to do with prognostic information. In order to translate prognosis into recommendation, we need to know about patient values" (Downar 2009, 168).

This concern, about values, was perhaps put best by Baruch Brody:

> Suppose that, with the help of a validated severity of illness scale, clinicians can accurately estimate the probability of the patient's surviving [the] current hospitalization if he or she receives all interventions available. Is that information as useful as it might seem initially? I think not. Patients who have a very poor probability of surviving their current hospitalization may still obtain through extensive medical interventions a prolongation of their life in the hospital before they die. This prolongation may be judged by them and/or their family to be of considerable significance.
>
> Conversely, patients who have a very high probability of surviving their current hospitalization through extensive interventions, but whose more long-term prognosis (even their six month survival rate) is extremely poor, may judge (or their families may judge for them) that the prolongation of life is of little significance compared to the heavy costs imposed by the extensive interventions. Clinicians who use severity of illness scales to determine the likelihood of survival for the current hospitalization, and who make judgments of futility or of utility on the basis of this likelihood, have chosen as their outcome-measure something that may not correspond either with their patient's values or with their own values. (Brody 1989, 663)

Tomorrow's scientific progress has a way of humbling (if not humiliating) yesterday's assurances. Prognostic scores can be drawn by the hour or day, and it develops that they are at their greatest accuracy in the short term. This means that if aggressive treatment might be able to get a patient past a certain point, the next score would improve. Moreover, as a general proposition, prediction models also seem to be of poor or questionable quality

(Collins et al. 2015). Further, APACHE-like systems are being joined, and perhaps superseded, by new generations of data-mining software such as artificial neural networks, support vector machines, and decision trees (Kim et al. 2011; cf. Moreno and Afonso 2006). The challenge here is, in part, to determine if they are more accurate, perhaps even asymptotically approaching some level of perfection, and, in larger part, to find a way to decide between or among them.

End-of-life care and the problem of "clinical futility"

There is a further problem. As it is, we collectively do a poor-to-mediocre job in communicating with patients about end-of-life issues. However, should we begin to try to incorporate information from computer scores in the patient-communication process? Indeed, it is likely we do not (Jennings 2006), thus undermining the valid-consent process.[20] The force of a report of clinical judgment ("I'm sorry, but I don't think you'll make it") is embedded in mass culture (it is one possible response to the earlier query "What are my chances, Doc?") and is strongly attached to the authority that accompanies judgments by trusted physicians and nurses. Contrarily, a computer score report ("I am sorry, but the computer has assigned your loved one a very low probability of survival; here are the multivariate physiological variables that were used in computing …") enjoys no such status.

In other words, patient and family naiveté and ignorance are the source of numerous existing problems in delivering bad news. Adding technological spin to such reports contributes little if anything to valid consent by patients or surrogates. Note that this is the case *even if the prognosis is perfectly and uncontroversially accurate*. At the end of life, being prognostically correct is itself not a sufficient condition for ethically maximized bedside manner and communication (cf. Brody 1989). Moreover, clinical truth telling requires more than numbers, even objective or accurate numbers, to be of value. This is one of the reasons some medical and nursing educators are wisely urged to refrain from the citation of statistics at the bedside. It will not be the case that prognostic scores will make a very difficult task – giving bad news – easier.

So now consider the possible value of a "computational futility index"[21] or a score generated by a prognostic scoring system that suggests that future treatment will fail according to one or more criteria under Stuart Youngner's (1988) well-known typology of clinical criteria:

- Physiological: e.g., when catecholamines do not increase blood pressure
- Postponing death: when intervention will not prolong life
- Length of life: when a life is saved, but only for a short while
- Quality of life: when life is prolonged but not improved
- Probability of success: when there is small chance of prolonging life, or prolonging life with quality

Here, in part, is how this was once parsed:

> What makes this typology useful is its demonstration that futility is not a global or monolithic concept, that decisions about further treatment must be relativized to goals (Youngner 1988). Additionally, there are rival models of physician obligations in futile or purportedly futile contexts (Jecker and Schneiderman 1993; Schneiderman and Jecker 1995). Under the weak model, physicians are free to withhold or discontinue futile efforts; a moderate obligation has it that physicians should be encouraged to withhold or discontinue futile

efforts; in the strong model, physicians must withhold or discontinue futile efforts. Each model has various strengths and weaknesses. What such a typology suggests is that there is much work to be done – independently of outcomes accuracy and prognostic scoring – before we can proclaim that a [computational futility index] provides support for terminating or withholding treatment (cf. Luce and Wachter 1994). This effort will occur in bioethics and related disciplines, where, it must be strongly emphasized, debates about futility are intense, multidisciplinary, and waged on many fronts. We have no uniform definition of futility, or even an agreement that one is needed.   (Goodman 1998c, 123)

This is still correct. It is not to suggest that a computational futility index is always inappropriate – just that it, alone, is inadequate to the task. If a hospital wanted to use prognostic scores as part of a comprehensive futility policy, it would be necessary to embed their use in a process that could be overruled or overridden by ethical, social, or other considerations. Then, for instance, any institutional response to a patient or family demanding that the team "do everything" to try to save a life should include an assessment of patient values, the accuracy of the score, and a review process, perhaps by an institutional ethics committee. That, in turn, will require that such committees be educated in biomedical informatics, a virtue also to be rewarded in cases not involving predictions of death:

Society's inability to come to terms with death, our collective denial of the dying process, and our refusal to acknowledge when the good fight should be abandoned – are [not] all due to a lack of objective *information*. It would be very nice if this were so. But it is not. We have had increasingly accurate information about outcomes for millennia. There is no shortage of evidence that many patients and/or surrogates are inclined to seek a full-court press against death, even in the absence of warrant to believe that it will do any good. The problem in each of these "do everything" cases is not a lack of objective information. It is rather a lack of education, a failure of communication, or a psychological inability to grasp when the game is lost. No [automated futility index], no objective mortality prediction, no computational line in the sand will accomplish what generations of families, physicians, nurses, and patients have failed to accomplish: a broad-based, mature, and realistic view of death and dying.   (Goodman 1996a, 115–6)

This should be read as a restatement of the fact that people practice medicine and nursing, and that these practices are not yet, and perhaps never will be, purely or exclusively, about the accurate rendering of diagnoses or prognoses.

Summing up: accountability, responsibility, and "learned intermediaries"

There is another way of putting this: When a computer advances clinical practice, we should use it. When a computer is all there is to clinical practice, then something will have gone terribly and sadly wrong.

This is not a sentiment – it is an attempt to shape and save a principle. Humans are responsible for the care of patients. The duties of accountability and responsibility are reviewed in detail in Chapters 4 and 6, but they matter here because we have introduced intelligent machines into the clinician–patient relationship. Indeed, we have become quite excited by the prospect, and computational decision making has long been a research program in its own right (see Berner 2007 for a review; Garg et al. 2005 and Kawamoto et al. 2005 for state-of-the-art appraisals; and Cohn 2013 for a popular account; cf. Goodman 2014). High rates of human misdiagnosis (Graber et al. 2012) make this a worthy scientific initiative.

In the law, the doctrine of the "learned intermediary" is instructive, to a point. Thus:

> [T]his doctrine provides that a manufacturer of a prescription drug or medical device fulfills, and consequently discharges, its duty to warn about a device's potentially harmful effects by providing warnings to the *physician* using the device. In other words, once the manufacturer has *adequately* warned the physicians of potential dangers of a device, the liability shifts from the manufacturer to the user-physician because it is the physician who makes the ultimate medical judgments regarding what course of action is to be followed. It also becomes the physician who is responsible for relaying the applicable warnings to his/her patients. This transfer of liability is justified on the grounds that products such as [computerized decision support systems (CDSS)] only serve to supplement and inform a physician's ultimate medical judgment which, in totality, is also based upon the physician's individualized knowledge of the patient, drug-susceptibilities, localized epidemiological concerns, and other relevant factors. Moreover, the learned intermediary doctrine permits vendors to escape liability under the presumption that physicians, nurses, pharmacists, and other health professionals should be able to identify and correct any errors generated by CDSS and are better suited to do so than the CDSS vendors who are closer to software programmers than practitioners of medicine.
>
> (Picciano and Goodman 2014, note omitted; original emphasis)

The concept of the learned intermediary is suggestive but not dispositive. As decision support systems increase in complexity, it does not make sense for an individual physician to become learned enough to serve as a computer's intermediary. Many people contribute to the development of a decision support system: designers, programmers, builders, documentation writers, and so on – hence known as the "problem of many hands" (Nissenbaum 1994). This magnifies the problem of responsibility, especially since something might have gone wrong anywhere. Certainly for some diagnoses and prognoses it would be strange for a clinician to allow herself to be trumped by a machine. But as a diagnosis or prognosis becomes more complex, it could then become irrational for her to dismiss the computer's advice. What is sorely wanted is for the decision support research community to explore not only human–machine comparisons but also studies in which humans are challenged to accept or reject a machine's advice. A clinician trained in nursing or medicine *and* in the use of a decision support system should not reflexively be blamed for accepting a faulty computational diagnosis (any more than she should be faulted for taking at face value an automatic cardiac pulse measurement delivered by a device presumed to be in good working order). Resolving this will also depend in part how far off plumb a machine's error actually is. A good clinician will and ought to catch at least some mistakes. Perhaps what is envisioned in the law is not a learned intermediary, but an infallible one.

The ethics chapter (Goodman et al. 2014) in the standard textbook in biomedical informatics (Shortliffe and Cimino 2014) has for several editions opened with this motto:

> *More and more the tendency is towards the use of mechanical aids to diagnosis; nevertheless, the five senses of the doctor do still, and must always, play the preponderating part in the examination of the sick patient. Careful observation can never be replaced by the tests of the laboratory. The good physician now or in the future will never be a diagnostic robot.* – Scottish surgeon Sir William Arbuthnot-Lane.   (Lane 1936)

It is a really good motto.

Notes

1. The recipe: "If the sperma, enclosed in a hermetically sealed glass, is buried in horse manure for about forty days, and properly 'magnetised' it begins to live and to move. After such a time it bears the form and resemblance of a human being, but it will be transparent and without a corpus. If it is now artificially fed with the *arcanum sanguinis hominis* [an *Arcanum* of human blood, or 'invisible fire, which destroys all diseases'] until it is about forty weeks old, and if allowed to remain during that time in the horse-manure in a continually equal temperature, it will grow into a human child, with all its members developed like any other child, such as could have been born by a woman; only it will be much smaller. We call such a being a homunculus, and it may be raised and educated like any other child, until it grows older and obtains reason and intellect, and is able to take care of itself. This is one of the greatest secrets, and it ought to remain a secret until the days approach when all secrets will be known" (Hartmann 1988, 174).

   The writer Pamela McCorduck, one of many who comes rightly to respect Paracelsus, "with his mad combination of swindle and science" (McCorduck 2004, 14), notes he also left instructions for his remains to be preserved in horse manure for 40 days so he could be resurrected, but one of his disciples "said the right spell at the wrong speed and ruined it all" (ibid.), obviously a variation from practice guidelines.

2. We return to this idea and theme in Chapter 5.

3. Paracelsus actually lived, practiced, and wrote, but as for the historical Hippocrates, famed as a physician, there is no document in the Hippocratic corpus that can actually be linked to him (Nutton 1996); his "writings" are thought to be the work of others, perhaps students or followers of Pythagoras.

   Regarding the humoral theory and other notes on the history of medicine, see for instance Clendening (1942). On the utility of phlebotomy, see Bulaj et al. (2000). The humoral theory is still accepted in some places (Flores and Quinlan 2014).

4. According to the WHO (www.who.int/classifications/icd/en/, accessed December 2014),

   > The International Classification of Diseases (ICD) is the standard diagnostic tool for epidemiology, health management and clinical purposes. This includes the analysis of the general health situation of population groups. It is used to monitor the incidence and prevalence of diseases and other health problems, proving a picture of the general health situation of countries and populations.
   >
   > ICD is used by physicians, nurses, other providers, researchers, health information managers and coders, health information technology workers, policy-makers, insurers and patient organizations to classify diseases and other health problems recorded on many types of health and vital records, including death certificates and health records. In addition to enabling the storage and retrieval of diagnostic information for clinical, epidemiological and quality purposes, these records also provide the basis for the compilation of national mortality and morbidity statistics by WHO Member States. Finally, ICD is used for reimbursement and resource allocation decision-making by some countries.

   The ICD is in its tenth formulation. Because of its importance for billing in the United States, and challenges in incorporating ICD codes into electronic records, the formal adoption of ICD-10 was at one point delayed by the US Department of Health and Human Services.

5. "SNOMED" is "Systematized Nomenclature of Medicine." See www.ihtsdo.org/snomed-ct/what-is-snomed-ct.

6. The name, however, appears to be that of a bar in Texas and a brand of motorcycle.

7. Isabel is a "diagnosis checklist tool to help clinicians broaden their differential diagnosis and recognize a disease at the point of care," cofounded by two parents after their child "was nearly fatally misdiagnosed" and which is often available through medical libraries (www.isabelhealthcare.com/home/default); note the proposed use of this tool with the now defunct "Google Glass." Visit www.mdcalc.com, for a vast repository of calculators, and www.symcat.com ("What is bothering you today?") for a patient-directed resource. The disclaimers attempt to make clear that these tools are for educational purposes. From MDCalc: "You went to medical school for a reason. Double-check your work, and trust your clinical judgment over a number or result. If the Glasgow Coma Scale comes out 14/15, but the patient's unarousable, which do you think is right? MDCalc cannot and will not be held legally, financially, or medically responsible for decisions made using its calculators, equations, and algorithms, and is for the use of medical professionals only." From Symcat: "This

tool is for educational purposes only. It is NOT intended for diagnostic purposes. Only a physician or licensed provider may diagnose and treat diseases."

Note also that concerns have been raised about conflicts of interest associated with some online decision support sites (Amber et al. 2014).

8. For other important early work see Szolovits and Pauker (1979) and de Dombal (1987).

9. Reminder system documentation stretches from McDonald (1976) and Duda and Shortliffe (1983) to Cleveringa et al. (2013) and Tenke et al. (2014). See Edworthy (2013) on alarm fatigue; and Menon et al. (2014) on losing track of clinical alerts. Embi and Leonard (2012) study the problem of fatigue resulting from alerts used to improve clinical trial recruitment.

10. Sometimes rendered as "computerized *provider* order entry systems" to capture the fact that nurses and other allied health professionals enjoy prescribing authority in some jurisdictions. That nurses capture most medication errors (Cho et al. 2014) could be an argument in support of expanding their prescribing authority. That CPOE systems generally reduce medication errors by physicians introduces the idea that some forms of health information technology might be considered as levers to expand the scope of practice for allied health professionals. We return to this issue later in this chapter.

11. In the course of writing this book I have collected reports of a number of such events. I have in each case asked for and received documentation, correspondence, or personal attestation. There is no doubt about the veracity of these accounts. It would be a worthy project for an informatics researcher, perhaps a Ph.D. student, or a journalist to collect all vendors' and/or manufacturers' policies on disclosure of such intellectual property. It is worth noting that in some cases, EHR vendor lawyers have threatened legal action for disclosure and in others internal institutional counsel, fearing litigation, have prevented disclosure. Many examples of the practice at issue are available on AMIA's "Implementation" Listserv (Implementation@lists.amia.org). For an introduction to some transparency-eroding practices, see Koppel and Kreda (2009) and Goodman et al. (2011). Many of these issues are taken up in Chapter 6, on "the e-health industry."

12. See www.healthit.gov/providers-professionals/achieve-meaningful-use/core-measures/drug-interaction-check, and the links therein.

13. It would be easy to cast this rendering as strident, naïve, or cranky. It is intended rather as an attempt to rank values, in the breach. Corporations do invest, or risk, large sums on speculation and in hopes of turning an honest profit. The point here (and elsewhere in this book) is not to begrudge the clever entrepreneur her due, but, rather, to insist that when it comes to health care, not all profits are what we have come to call "revenue neutral." That is, if the cost of the profit is diminished patient safety, reduced public health, or increased disparity, then other values must be brought to bear. There is at the end of the day, or the end of time, only so much wealth honorably to be acquired from the misfortunes of sick people.

14. In part because of this, the US Institute of Medicine's Health Care Quality Initiative, which has included the reports *To Err Is Human: Building a Safer Health System* and *Crossing the Quality Chasm: A New Health System for the 21st Century*, is conducting a consensus study, "Diagnostic Error in Health Care."

15. In addition, there are powerful social and legal forces at play here. Humans and not computers are educated, licensed, and accredited for clinical practice (Goodman et al. 2014). It is difficult to imagine a change in this custom, meaning that for the foreseeable future, humans and human responsibility must be assumed to have a controlling role. A discussion of the law's "learned intermediary" doctrine in a related context follows.

16. The traditional distinction between "education" to increase knowledge and improve critical thinking and "training" to teach skills is often neglected, and the terms are often and unfortunately used interchangeably. Generally, I mean to be suggesting that both education and correlate training are required for the purposes here. Moreover, while training can be episodic and a skill thereby acquired can remain valid in the absence of additional training, those whose work affects human well-being requires ongoing, indeed, lifelong, education. The problem for many of our institutions is that the need to document change entails the practical supremacy of training. It is easier to document skill acquisition than an increase in knowledge, understanding, or critical thinking. This, in conjunction with attempts to reduce conflict-mediated corruption of medical learning, has led to the unhappy preeminence of measurable *behavior* change in continuing medical education.

17.   One important consideration is the validity, scope, and fitness for purpose of any particular diagnostic system. It has been pointed out that most computerized decision support systems have been used and evaluated in the context of internal medicine, and that specialties have "unique needs" (McCoy et al. 2013).

18.   Farr founded and edited the weekly journal *British Annals of Medicine, Pharmacy, Vital Statistics and General Science*, which survived only eight months, but was succeeded by others. It was apparently the first journal to use vital statistics, a practice then emulated by *The Lancet* and *British Medical Journal*: "Farr began to work on the statistical studies of English life tables used by insurance actuaries. He regarded a life table as a *biometer,* because it gave the 'exact measure of the duration of life under given circumstances' " (Magnello 2011, 270).

19.   In the first elaboration of the acronym, "we choose to stand for the system's major components – acute physiology, age, and chronic health evaluation" (Knaus et al. 1981). How "age" became "and" is anecdotally reported to be the result of recognition that age itself was a poor outcome predictor, an important point for teachers of end-of-life care.

   Apache Medical Systems, Inc., was sold in 2001 to one of the world's largest manufacturers of electronic health records, which reports that "APACHE is the most widely utilized clinical prediction tool among adult ICUs for evaluating expected outcomes such as: length of stay, mortality, ventilator days and need for active treatment." See www.cerner.com/cerner_research_shows_how_apache_outcomes_properly_analyzes_icu_performance_for_benchmarking/, and Knaus (2002) for an account of the creation of APACHE's intellectual property and the opposition that elicited.

20.   Jennings here also protests,

   To maintain jurisdiction over the care of patients, physicians share the data with the payers and regulators of care to prove they are using resources effectively and efficiently, yet they use the system in conjunction with moral principles to justify treating each patient as unique. Thus, concern for the individual patient is not lessened with the use of this system. However, physicians do not share the data with patients or surrogate decision-makers because they fear they will be viewed as more interested in profits than patients.

21.   As originally proposed, it was called a "computational futility metric" (Goodman 1996a); cf. Goodman (1998a, from which this chapter borrows in small part).

Health privacy, data protection, and trust

3

Hippocrates' "sacred secrets" are undiminished in importance in a world of electronic health records and cloud storage of vast amounts of personal data and information. Privacy and confidentiality are no less important to patients now than when information was stored in sheaves of paper in binders in racks at the foot of hospital beds. What has changed is that clinicians have increasingly complex duties to safeguard patient information, patients have more rights and opportunities to review it, and our ability to use that information to benefit others has never been greater. Privacy was never a right to be conferred or enjoyed in isolation from other entitlements and duties. Privacy and confidentiality are precious – but not absolute. "Sensitive information" raises the stakes, but appropriate governance strategies can help provide practical solutions. The creation and use of unique patient identifiers pose new challenges, but offer significant benefits.

Privacy and its foundations

Many years ago, a medical student showed up with a disheveled stack of pages that were wrinkled and dirty and therefore could not easily have their edges lined up the way one would when a sheaf is tapped on a desk. He had seen them fluttering in the street and snatched one to have a look. It was clearly a page from a medical record – and so he set about collecting as many as he could. It was a windy day.

The student wanted advice about what to do next.

In the daily grind, health professionals embody or reflect personal stances to information about their patients. They take privacy more or less seriously and, when challenged, go to different lengths to protect it. Many of these professionals have been to the privacy and confidentiality workshop or orientation where, in the United States, the discussion overwhelmingly, if not exclusively, turned on provisions of the Privacy Rule under the Health Insurance Portability and Accountability Act, or HIPAA. In Europe, learners are taught about Data Protection Directive 95/46/EC and perhaps the forthcoming General Data Protection Regulation. In the United Kingdom they are taught about the Data Protection Act, the advent of Summary Care Records, and the Human Rights Act.[1] That is, health professionals are told what privacy laws govern their behavior. In the United States, at least, the workshops sometimes tend to include stern warning about fines and other punishments for "noncompliance" or other violations. While HIPAA calls for institutions to appoint a privacy officer, this is often a compliance officer or located in a compliance office.

This is all to say that in many respects, the role of privacy education and privacy protection in contemporary health care has been assigned to general counsel, compliance, and risk management offices. That is not a bad thing in itself, but it can or does entail that the moral foundations of rights to privacy – the *reasons* why we value and protect it – are decoupled from daily professional practice. The relationship between privacy and other values is not elucidated, and the strategies for resolving conflicts among those values are left unaddressed. The idea that professionals behave a certain way because it is the right way, and not because they will otherwise be punished, is not reinforced.

This chapter reviews some of the moral foundations of privacy and confidentiality, identifies places where conflict arises and how to resolve it, and addresses some of the compromises to be entertained when other values have legitimate claims to predominance. Some of the rights and responsibilities will be seen to be ancient and some to arise in an e-health world. At ground, health information is reckoned to be special – extra sensitive, more reflective of vulnerability, and a greater source of fear than most or all other forms of personal information.

It should be emphasized that "privacy" and "confidentiality" are not synonyms. Generally, "confidentiality" applies to information, whereas "privacy" applies to individual people and should be understood to include, more broadly, their concerns about confidentiality, as well as their desire not to be the target of various forms of eavesdropping. Suppose someone follows you and repeatedly observes you entering an HIV/AIDS clinic;[2] we might say then your privacy has been violated. If someone else sneaks into the clinic without seeing you and looks at your electronic health record, the record's confidentiality has been breached (Goodman et al. 2014). Regarding electronic health records, "privacy" may also refer to the desire to limit personal data disclosure (National Research Council 1997).

The student who had scrambled in the street to collect the wayward paper records later learned that a file had somehow fallen from a briefcase, and the pages were returned to the clinician who had made the mistake of removing them from the office in the first place. I congratulated the student for doing something he was not required by any law to do, for someone he did not know, and for acting without knowledge of any bad consequences that might otherwise result. He blushed, then shrugged.

Privacy and confidentiality are ancient values. Although we count them now as rights, it is likely that their first articulations were not motivated by philosophical considerations of human or civil rights but, rather, by narrowly practical considerations. Our infirmities distress and sometimes embarrass us. They can be difficult to talk about and often challenge inter- and transcultural taboos related to communicating about sickness and sexuality, digestion and death. But if something is difficult to talk about, and a physician or nurse is the interlocutor, then that clinician might not hear the full story, or even enough of the story to begin her work on a diagnosis and treatment plan. If, further, there is any risk that a clinician might share the story, then the unhappy patient is incentivized to speak less than candidly and less than truthfully. Patients lie, and this obstructs clinical practice. Hippocrates understood this and rendered it a rule: "Whatsoever in the course of practice I see or hear (or even outside my practice in social intercourse) that ought never to be published abroad, I will not divulge, but consider such things to be holy secrets" (BMJ 1998, 1110).[3] This was not the result of complex analysis, but the distillation of experience.

What is more, this insight has enjoyed some 2,400 years of professional uptake and now enjoys special status in all health practices. This point cannot be emphasized enough: The concern for privacy and confidentiality is *internal* to these professions. Medical privacy was invented by doctors – not contemporary lawyers, risk managers, or compliance officials, not legislatures, policy makers or philosophers – though it is true that physicians have ceded this and other moral authority too often and too easily. This has led some to believe that privacy and data protection are barriers and impediments to clinical practice and research. This, too, is a mistake.

It is also a great pity, especially given that we are now not talking about lambskin or papyrus scrolls, but electronic health records, Big Data, and the clouds that contain them. In addition to the traditional and practical value of keeping confidences, there are strong and broader grounds to do so.

This has been repeatedly recognized, as has the fact that a right not protected by law might not be much of a right. In "The Right to Privacy," Samuel Warren and Louis Brandeis, who would later be a US Supreme Court justice, grounded privacy rights in antecedently recognized rights to free expression ("no fixed formula can be used to prohibit obnoxious publications" Warren and Brandeis 1890, 215), concluding that:

> It would doubtless be desirable that the privacy of the individual should receive the added protection of the criminal law, but for this, legislation would be required. Perhaps it would be deemed proper to bring the criminal liability for such publication within narrower limits; but that the community has an interest in preventing such invasions of privacy, sufficiently strong to justify the introduction of such a remedy, cannot be doubted. Still, the protection of society must come mainly through a recognition of the rights of the individual. Each man is responsible for his own acts and omissions only. If he condones what he reprobates, with a weapon at hand equal to his defense, he is responsible for the results. If he resists, public opinion will rally to his support. Has he then such a weapon? It is believed that the common law provides him with one, forged in the slow fire of the centuries, and to-day fitly tempered to his hand. The common law has always recognized a man's house as his castle, impregnable, often, even to his own officers engaged in the execution of its command. Shall the courts thus close the front entrance to constituted authority, and open wide the back door to idle or prurient curiosity? (ibid., 219–20)[4]

Privacy is wound so tightly into the fabric of most human life that it is easily overlooked. Indeed and however, the unthinking assumption that some things should be kept private helps underpin basic freedoms to enjoy solitude, to exercise autonomy, to be individuals. Privacy is a means for controlling which parts of our lives are to be shared with or known to others (Alpert 1995, 1998). Alpert identifies key and insightful analyses of the foundation for privacy rights. Thus, in brief, privacy:

- is "based on the idea that there is a close connection between our ability to control who has access to us and to information about us, and our ability to create and maintain different sorts of social relationships with different people" (Rachels 1975, 292).
- "[d]enotes a degree of inaccessibility of persons, of their mental states, and of information about them to the senses and surveillance devices of others" (Allen 1988, 3).
- is related to "the extent to which we are known to others [secrecy], the extent to which others have physical access to us [solitude], and the extent to which we are the subject of others' attention [anonymity]. [Privacy matters] because of our anonymity, because no one is interested in us. The moment someone becomes sufficiently interested, he may find it quite easy to take all that privacy away" (Gavison 1984, 379).
- is "fundamental to respect, love, friendship, and trust; indeed, some argue, without privacy these relationships are inconceivable" (Alpert 1998, citing Fried 1968).

Ensuring privacy thus emerges not as an act of kindness or courtesy, not as a surrender to shyness or embarrassment, and not as troublesome impediment to our keen desires to know juicy bits about others' lives. It emerges as a human entitlement, without which life as we know it would not be possible. As other entitlements, including health care and public health, however, it is not, cannot, and ought not to be absolute.

Tools for protecting privacy and confidentiality

The challenge before us is in many respects independent of the media in which personal health information is stored, that is, whether the information is kept on paper or electronically. It is a long-standing challenge, and it is this: What is the best way to make the information very easily available to those who need and ought to have it (including patients themselves), and very difficult for those who do not need and ought not to have it?

> All health care information systems, whether paper or computer, present confidentiality and privacy problems ... Computerization can reduce some concerns about privacy in patient data and worsen others, but it also raises new problems. Computerization increases the quantity and availability of data and enhances the ability to link the data, raising concerns about new demands for information beyond those for which it was originally collected. The potential for abuse of privacy by trusted insiders to a system is of particular concern.
>
> (OTA 1993a, 3; cf. OTA 1993b)

Here are the two extremes between which we need to find a middle ground that is flexible and responsive to the needs of patients, caregivers, and public health. At the one extreme is the *ubiquitous access*: Imagine that everyone's medical records, histories, and information are stored on the Superdupercloud, available to anyone who wants to have a look. Look up your neighbor, friend, or intimate partner to see the full record; check on your favorite actor or football player or colleague (or even those who are not favorites); or just browse through the records of strangers in the hope of deriving some comfort from the comparison. At the other extreme is the *anonotronics approach*: No information is ever stored anywhere and, indeed, clinicians are forbidden from making any kind of note at all about any patient encounter. Vital statistics records are not kept.

We see potential and partial exemplars of the former in cases of very large data breaches in which patient records are disclosed, when they are either accidently published, hacked, or stored on media later stolen.[5] The latter is partly exemplified every time a patient pays cash and requests that his information not be shared, as for instance with a health plan, or, better, when patients pay out of pocket and give a false name.

In any case, it is uncontroversial that neither option makes sense medically, socially, or ethically. What is wanted is a trustworthy and secure system that supports the collection and storage of information – lots of information – and makes it available only when appropriate. There are several reasons why this is exquisitely difficult. Three are most salient, and their inter-relations are complex.

The first is social. One of the reasons some people are worried about access to their health information is that in some jurisdictions it can be used for various forms of discrimination, including access to health care itself. In the United States, for instance, it was once legal for insurance companies to deny coverage to patients for "pre-existing conditions," a stratagem to justify the denial of health care to people because they are sick. Medically preposterous and ethically illegitimate, the practice was eliminated by the Affordable Care Act or "Obamacare" in 2014.[6] Similarly, the 2008 Genetic Insurance Nondiscrimination Act (GINA) prohibits insurance or employment discrimination based on genetic information.[7] More significantly, however, are the challenges posed by stigma, bias, and forms of "soft discrimination." If health information somehow leaks from the clinic to … well, anywhere, then a patient might fear ostracism, neglect, or other forms of social disapprobation. This social element is both well known and difficult to document. The scope of "appropriate" disclosure can be equally difficult to plot.

The next difficulty in crafting a trusted and secure health information system is political. Here is a hypothesis: Most ordinary people value privacy, but also the benefits that come from the responsible use of their information, including research, public health surveillance, outcome analysis, quality improvement, and so on; we could even cast those values as legitimate rights, too, such as, a right to a sound public health infrastructure, a right to evidence-based health care, and so on. This way, a valuable right is balanced by another valuable right. Moreover, these ordinary people understand they cannot be asked individually for each such legitimate use of their information. This is a testable hypothesis. At ground, the political challenge consists in balancing individual rights with collective goods, an issue we return to in Chapter 8, on research and public health. One is not a "privacy opponent" because she values public health. Unfortunately, examples of patients being so fearful of information disclosure that they restricted their own access to health care have fueled the engines of "privacy advocates," so-called because of their uncompromising stance regarding the scope of permissible uses of information collected during clinical and hospital encounters.

The third is ethics, or value-based analysis of positions and propositions articulated either from first principles or during social or political debates. As we will see in Chapter 6, even legislative debates might actually be about ethics and values, though they are often, as such, of disappointing quality. Neither Utilitarianism nor a rights-based approach alone is adequate to resolve the delicate balancing issue at hand (cf. Angst 2009). What is required is a series of arguments and counterarguments with the best answer being that which maximizes utility, or benefits, to the population, and minimizes any limitation on rights. Something like this will be required if we are to derive the greatest benefit and least harm and wrong from cloud data storage. Absolutists or purists will find little succor here. It is, moreover, an unfortunate fact of contemporary life that even in open societies, sometimes, the best solution is not accepted, or adopted, by legislatures and policy makers.

We should linger here briefly. Utilitarianism, or the maximizing of collective goods, can range over individual actions or over a series of acts of following a rule. Rule Utilitarianism manages counterexamples such as an Act Utilitarian abridgement of minority rights in exchange for majority benefit. In many cases, and especially for public health, Utilitarianism wins. It would be perverse to suggest, for instance, that an Ebola patient not lose the liberty to move about freely or, more importantly here, that his diagnosis not be shared with any who are tasked with finding, transporting, or caring for him; the same might be said about a floridly psychotic patient who poses a risk to others. This is not to say that their information can be slung about willy-nilly, only that there are several well-motivated exceptions to standard and equally well-motivated privacy-protection rules. The psychiatry patient who pays in cash out of fear of stigma or bias is poorly served by enacting laws to make it more difficult for researchers to analyze data about him or for his future hospitals to treat him. As we saw, moreover, there are also very strong Utilitarian reasons to protect privacy. Rights-and-duties-based accounts, or Kantian or deontological theories, to be useful in public policy, must carefully identify and motivate exceptions to the exercise of rights in addition to identifying the rights themselves. It is for this reason that the practice of law, the writing of sound legislation, and the exercise of wise jurisprudence can be so difficult.

At the intersection of the social, the political, and the ethical lie strategies, mechanisms, and tools to accommodate the first, manage the second, and honor the last. These strategies, mechanisms, and tools may be used at the level of individual practices as well as by legislative authorities. I am here most interested in *education, policies,* and *technology itself* (cf. Alpert 1993, 1998).

Recall from Chapter 2 the argument that education is an ethical imperative or obligation for health professionals. That argument serves us well here. The idea is simple, and, more or less, this: Ordinary health professionals and researchers (a subset of the ones we just appealed to understand that it is ethically straightforward to regard privacy as a right that must be balanced against other rights) do not generally want, intend, or plan to breach their patients' confidentiality. Indeed, they likely value it for themselves. A curriculum that makes clear (i) that and how common morality requires attention to privacy and confidentiality; (ii) the practical steps for accomplishing this; and (iii) that there are mechanisms in place to ensure these protections then becomes an essential step in the privacy and confidentiality protection effort. It is here that we teach that health information is special, its disclosure can wrong people, and that protecting it increases the chances for good outcomes. This curriculum is expected to describe the institutional policies that guide and govern behavior. It should also explain how audit trails keep dynamic track of all electronic record system users' access to patient records, better to identify employees who inappropriately view those records (no, you are not permitted to look up the chart of the gentleman dating your sister after you think you glimpse him at the infectious disease clinic).

"Policies" here refers to both institutional policies and public policies or laws. These policies lay out who may legitimately access patient records, and when. They make clear whether and when valid consent is required from patients to examine their information. Policies should address the use of e-mail and the question whether students may view the records of last week's patients. Consider in this regard the "minimum necessary requirement" under US privacy law:

> The minimum necessary standard, a key protection of the HIPAA Privacy Rule, is derived from confidentiality codes and practices in common use today. It is based on sound current practice that protected health information should not be used or disclosed when it is not necessary to satisfy a particular purpose or carry out a function. The minimum necessary standard requires covered entities to evaluate their practices and enhance safeguards as needed to limit unnecessary or inappropriate access to and disclosure of protected health information. The Privacy Rule's requirements for minimum necessary are designed to be sufficiently flexible to accommodate the various circumstances of any covered entity.

Moreover:

> For uses of protected health information, the covered entity's policies and procedures must identify the persons or classes of persons within the covered entity who need access to the information to carry out their job duties, the categories or types of protected health information needed, and conditions appropriate to such access. For example, hospitals may implement policies that permit doctors, nurses, or others involved in treatment to have access to the entire medical record, as needed. Case-by-case review of each use is not required. Where the entire medical record is necessary, the covered entity's policies and procedures must state so explicitly and include a justification. For routine or recurring

requests and disclosures, the policies and procedures may be standard protocols and must limit the protected health information disclosed or requested to that which is the minimum necessary for that particular type of disclosure or request.[8]

Notice the tacit appeal to the ethics of "confidentiality codes" and the need for flexibility. This law, the first nationwide effort to address privacy and confidentiality, its predecessors being laws for each individual state, strives to achieve the elusive goal we began with, that is, to make access difficult for those who ought not to have it, and easy for those who ought. Whether it has succeeded or not is a topic of ongoing debate (Bilimoria 2009; Lane and Schur 2010).

The third tool, in addition to education and sound policy, is technological. Make it difficult to violate privacy and breach confidentiality. This requires powerful ways to protect from external threats to data and strong security measures to thwart "trusted insiders," or those, perhaps with internal credentials, who attempt unauthorized access to patient records. Audit trails provide one kind of protection, nimble authentication protocols another. Getting this right is extremely difficult, in part because barriers to inappropriate use can also impede appropriate use. Privacy protection can be built into system design, embodying the principles of privacy-enhancing technologies and "privacy by design" (Hustinx 2010).[9] Even here, however, there is no universal agreement on best practices. If the devil is in the details, then this is a particularly malevolent evil spirit, and there are a great many details. Such complexity helps to shape the tight link between policies and security:

> Data protection policies, if they are to be effective in this rapidly changing environment, must not be tied to specific systems and system capabilities but, rather, must establish security protection guidelines that define system goals but do not specify how these goals will be reached. These protections will be most effective if privacy is addressed directly at the outset in developing electronic systems. (Gostin et al. 1993, 2491)

One significant effort is based on data protection standards developed by Health Level 7 International (HL7), the leading standards development organization, which has published code sets "specifying the security classification of acts and roles in accordance with the definition for concept domain 'confidentiality.'" There are six levels of security ranging from "unrestricted" to "very restricted."[10] The role of security standards cannot be overemphasized; the broader scope of standards in health information technology is addressed in Chapter 5.

These three gears – education, policies, and technology – must mesh to drive the privacy engine. Education, policy, and technology/security are interlocking requirements such that if any one of them is of low quality or insincere or lacks thoughtfulness, then patient information will be inadequately protected. There is a lot of work that remains to be done, and we will have failed if education focuses on fines, institutional policies are purchased from consultants, and IT units are not run by professionals.

"Sensitive information," compromise, and governance

There is a lot to like in the recognition that patients have a special relationship to information about them. This entails many things, not least that patients should easily be able to access and review that information, as discussed in Chapter 1, where we recalled the days in which patients were not permitted to receive copies of their own health records. There was no reason for this – it was a patronizing and ad hoc stance adopted by the keepers of patient records. One can imagine several motivations for such a practice, perhaps the best being the belief that the more information hidden in this way, the less likelihood of losing a lawsuit. There is little or no basis for such a belief.

It is more than 40 years since the United States' Fair Trade Commission published its guidelines for "fair information practices" (US Department of Health, Education and Welfare 1973), which, correctly, begins, "Computers linked together through high-speed telecommunications networks are destined to become the principal medium for making, storing, and using records about people. Innovations now being discussed throughout government and private industry recognize that the computer-based record, keeping system, if properly used, can be a powerful management tool." In 1980, the Council of Europe ratified the Convention for the Protection of Individuals with regard to Automatic Processing of Personal Data, the antecedent of all subsequent European Union data protection legislation. ("The purpose of this convention is to secure in the territory of each Party for every individual, whatever his nationality or residence, respect for his rights and fundamental freedoms, and in particular his right to privacy, with regard to automatic processing of personal data relating to him ('data protection')" (Council of Europe 1981).)

Fair information practices include provisions for notice (or "awareness") so that data collectors, uses, and users are identified. Thereafter, data sources should in principle be able to opt in or opt out of those uses. The overarching motivation for this and subsequent legislation is to establish and sustain trust in the people whose data is being collected and used – even if it is being done so for their sake. Thus:

> At its core, HIPAA embodies the idea that individuals should have access to their own health data, and more control over uses and disclosures of that health data by others. Among its provisions, the law requires that patients be informed about their privacy rights, including a right of access; that uses and disclosures of "protected health information" generally be limited to exchanges of the "minimum necessary"; that uses and disclosures for other than treatment, payment and health care operations be subject to patient authorization; and that all employees in "covered entities" (institutions that HIPAA legally affects) be educated about privacy and information security.   (Goodman et al. 2014, 349)[11]

Not incongruently, the EU Data Protection Directive requires that data be:

> collected for specified, explicit and legitimate purposes and not further processed in a way incompatible with those purposes. Further processing of data for historical, statistical or scientific purposes shall not be considered as incompatible provided that Member States provide appropriate safeguards ...[12]

But identifying principles and legislating their formal adoption is an ongoing and, indeed, never-ending task. There will never come the day when we complete this effort, dust our hands, and stride off confidently in search of new challenges. Since the birth of HIPAA, a refined set of principles makes clear that many public benefits result from the careful and transparent use of data and information, for instance, "Access to and use of health data should be viewed as a public good. Data should be available and 'fit-for-use', with proper security, for appropriate purposes beyond direct patient care" (Hripcsak et al. 2014).

This is deceptively simple to state, and exquisitely difficult to achieve. Let us assume for the sake of discussion that we will soon enter an era in which wise education, sound policy, and strict security conjointly and successfully manage the most common threats to privacy and confidentiality, namely, intrusions by hackers, "sightseeing" by trusted insiders, and inappropriate record access driven by what we might call "scope creep" or access beyond role.

Now it gets really interesting. Some of the privacy and confidentiality challenges generated by electronic health records and the sharing of their information, as among health information exchanges, resemble challenges from paper records; others are created or magnified by the tools of information technology. Meeting these challenges will test the ability of applied ethics to be of nontrivial and practical use.

Behavioral, sexual, and genetic "exceptionalism"

The schizophrenic with HIV/AIDS and a p53 mutation will likely have a difficult life, though some of the worst of his difficulties will be shaped or even created by society. What is sensitive here today might not be sensitive there tomorrow. Besides, any illness or injury can in principle be embarrassing. Some people, perhaps many, perhaps even most, depending on the culture, will, in one degree or another, be biased against, think less of, stigmatize others, and otherwise hold them in diminished regard, especially if they have certain kinds of maladies. The best-studied diseases in the social science literature seem to be those related to behavioral, sexual, and genetic health, though stigma also accompanies non-sexually transmitted infectious diseases, including leprosy and maladies related to hygiene. Epilepsy can be stigmatizing, also obesity and amblyopia. Ebola, smoking, and many ordinary bodily functions are sometimes stigmatizing, and even birth defects, several gastrointestinal disorders, and severe acne. Cancer can be stigmatizing, and so is heart disease, especially for smokers. Disability can be stigmatizing. Death, too. It is a long list, a sad catalogue of human ignorance, cruelty, and stupidity.[13]

Alas, 'twas ever thus. Although fear of stigma and discrimination amplify privacy concerns, surely the instruments of health information technology cannot be responsible for eliminating or mitigating the variable, cultural, and often ugly responses to disease, most of which have existed in one form or another for millennia.

Equally surely, those instruments ought not to make it worse. In the best possible world, health information technology might actually *improve* widely valued protections. So, for instance, in the early days of HIV/AIDS, many institutions and jurisdictions created or required specially sequestered parts of the health record to bolster trust in their confidentiality to encourage people to be tested for the virus. Such partitioning, to prevent or impede inappropriate access while maintaining access facility for those who need it, can be better achieved electronically than in a paper chart.

Generally, though, there should be a very good reason to create a unique protection for any particular kind of health information, lest those without the malady that enjoys special protection have warrant to allege discrimination against them or *their* malady. Public health provides one such reason. Moreover, if and when the stigma storm dissipates, any special protection should be removed. Most importantly, if a society contributes to or fosters stigma and discrimination, perhaps by having an inadequate health system, then the best solution is to fix the health system – not to create jerry-rigged security protocols that give special status to particular maladies. A virtue of the approach to privacy taken here – that all health information should enjoy confidentiality protections – means that patients should not have to make the case or argue for their particular malady or source of embarrassment or fount of discrimination and stigma. In principle, information about my stubbed toe should receive the same protection as my HIV status or depression diagnosis.

That said, genetic information poses distinctive problems in virtue of the fact that a person's genetic information is also, in one degree or another, information about others as well. A genetic datum about a mother might have significance to her daughter, or vice versa. One feature of a datum's significance is that it might be that someone does not want to know about it – as, for instance, in the case of genetic maladies for which there is no treatment. Moreover, we are very close to the day when routine testing will regularly reveal surprises in the family tree related to paternity, adoption, and consanguinity. These are all well-known challenges in the ethics-and-genetics literature. They are now, or eventually will be, problems for the electronic storage and analysis of genomic and genetic information.

A delicious sin, which many of us are guilty of enjoying, is what might be called "problem lensing" or "dilemma savoring." By this I mean the inclination to sketch an ethical challenge, issue, or problem, make it seem very worrisome, and then declare it to be an intractable dilemma worthy of sustained hand-wringing: "Lo, an ethical dilemma!" The worried attention devoted to the publication in 2013 of a fascinating report in which individual surnames could be identified from computational analyses of shared and (otherwise) unidentified sequence sets is a good example of grist for the dilemma-savoring mill:

> This study shows that data release, even of a few markers, from one person can spread through deep genealogical ties and lead to the identification of another person who might have no acquaintance with the person who released his genetic data. The propagation of information through shared male lines amplifies the range of identification, allowing ~135,000 records to potentially target several million U.S. males. Another feature of this identification technique is that it entirely relies on free, publicly available resources. It can be completed end-to-end with only computational tools and an Internet connection.
>
> (Gymrek et al. 2013, 324)

Although this poses challenges for biomedical research, which are addressed in Chapter 8, it is worrisome to suppose such cleverness has identified a problem to be solved before we can securely reap the benefits of genomic practice. If global and airtight protections against re-identifying biological samples, or people, are required to realize the benefits of genetic research, then such research will be impossible.

In any case, we had enough problems on our plate before this. Consider the challenges posed by parental access to their children's electronic health records and the protection of sensitive parental information that might be in those records (Bayer et al. 2015). To address this successfully will require a suite of compromise and rights-balancing skills: generally, compromise when possible, and, when not possible, have in place sound structures for conflict management and resolution.

In fact, a readily available and rapidly improving tool for both clinical practice and research, including translational research, is that of trusted governance systems or processes (Kaye 2012). Under trusted (sometimes "honest") governance, data are collected, stored, analyzed, and shared under public policies and protocols that identify security protections, policies for appropriate uses and users, risks, sharing partners, and so on. The databases are constantly being analyzed for quality, care, and research. Atop this structure is a group of people appointed to monitor the enterprise and, especially, make judgments about how to manage and communicate incidental findings, requested exceptions to prior rules, and special cases. (Patient Zeta has just been found to have been exposed to prions during neurosurgery; should he be informed? If so, by whom?) We return to this issue in Chapter 8.

Trusted governance does not need to be perfect or infallible. That should perhaps be obvious, but our institutions and policies too often are inclined to make the perfect the enemy of the good. There are no credible current guarantees that Neptunian terrorists will not hack your record and publish your embarrassing diseases on the Web, but the absence of such a guarantee would be a poor reason not to seek health care or allow your physicians and nurses to maintain accurate and comprehensive records. Our management of information about behavioral maladies, sexually transmitted diseases, and genetics and heritable disorders must be advanced in a similarly nimble way, that is, with a process that respects core values, is transparent, governed by thoughtful citizens, and accountable to the community it purports to serve.

We should conceive here of the creation of analogues to hospital ethics committees. These committees, at their best, have reduced liability and conflict, kept cases out of court, and engendered trust. Imperfect in many respects, they nevertheless help in the management of some of our most difficult problems. Indeed, the fact that very few ethics committees address issues in digital health, and very few in the world of biomedical informatics would consider turning to them, suggests a suite of fertile opportunities for collaboration and research (Goodman 1999).

Patient X: unique identifiers for health care

Just earlier we brushed against the issue of de- and re-identification of health care information. In fact, every patient's electronic health record is unique, and any comprehensive and robust system to analyze these records can in principle link a data set with an individual person. In other words, with enough information, it is possible to find or identify an individual in a large group. Absent the kinds of controls and oversight mulled here, such a re-identification might constitute a violation of privacy. It is simultaneously a means of improving patient safety, care delivery and outcomes, practical hospital epidemiology, public health surveillance, biomedical research, and so on. We also know that the problem of de- and re-identifying data and information is "among the most interesting, difficult and important in all health computing" (Goodman et al. 2014, 339; cf. also the references therein, especially Atreya et al. 2013; Benitez and Malin 2010; Malin and Sweeney 2004; Malin et al. 2011; Sweeney 1997; Tamersoy et al. 2012).

This tension between an ordinary and useful tool – the unique patient identifier – and risks to privacy and confidentiality warrants scrutiny.

While it is true that a unique identifier would make it easier to find a particular individual and, in principle, allow a malicious person to do various kinds of mischief, surely that alone cannot constitute sufficient warrant to disdain the creation and use of such an identifier for health care. There are several reasons for this. One is that we are already associated with or linked to a variety of more-or-less unique identifiers ranging from e-mail addresses to credit card numbers. It is a striking and never-ending source of amazement that some people – often fancied to be "privacy advocates" – will abjure uses of and risks from a unique health identifier while cheerily allowing banks, retail vendors, online click-stream sniffers, credit card companies, and others to make free with their personal information. Ubiquitous tracking of personal financial data is embraced in exchange for ease in buying bric-a-brac or concert tickets on the Web, while legitimate use of health data to track disease and improve health care delivery is somehow reckoned to pose utterly unacceptable risks. Further, in the United States, the Social Security number, intended as a unique national identifier, has come to be used widely in health care despite many shortcomings, not least that many people do not have one and, in some circumstances, two or more persons share one. At any rate, people have become used to free transmission of that number or sections of it for health care and other purposes. Another reason in support of unique identifiers is larger and too-infrequently recognized: There is actually very little evidence in support of the notion that ordinary people are willing to trade improved health care for stricter data-protection policies and, indeed, they actually *assume and prefer* that appropriate use is being made of their personal information without explicit consent (Marquard and Brennan 2009; Meslin and Goodman 2010).

A great assumption of public policy – that patients value privacy and confidentiality above all else – seems to have been woven from the most slender of threads.[14]

Searching for balance

At the least, in the absence of a unique identifier, there is an urgent need to do a better job matching various records with patients and patients with their records. In the United States, a report commissioned by the Office of the National Coordinator for Health Information Technology made a strong case for better identification and matching:

> Driven by concerns for patient safety in the event of mismatched or unmatched records and the national imperative to improve population health and lower costs through care coordination, this initiative studied both technical and human processes, seeking improvements to patient identification and matching that could be quickly implemented and lead to near-term improvements in matching rates. The findings presented in this report have been developed with the participation of healthcare stakeholders across many sectors and a wide geography. Lessons were drawn from individuals and organizations working to improve patient identification and matching on the bleeding edge of technology, as well as from those taking a systematic approach to improving data quality within the technical systems storing patient data, through review and rework of business processes. The combination of those approaches has contributed to findings that suggest the standardization of specific demographic fields within health information systems, broad collaboration on industry best practices that could both inform policy and be shared nationally, and areas for further study where additional advances could be made in the future. (Morris et al. 2014)[15]

A useful distinction, which might help clear the path, is between and among risks, harms, and wrongs (Goodman and Prineas 2009), where the distinction is a tool for sorting out questions in biomedical research. For our purposes here, there is and will always be *risks* of privacy violations and confidentiality breaches. However, it is the duty of information stewards to minimize those risks. When a risk, always probabilistic, is realized it becomes a harm or wrong. To be *harmed* by a privacy violation or confidentiality breach would require that an individual come to grief in one way or another, perhaps by suffering embarrassment or stigma, by enduring bias or discrimination, or by losing or forfeiting some benefit. It is also possible that a risk is realized, but the party at risk does not know it; it might, for instance, be that a health record is lost, released, or otherwise compromised, but no harm comes of it. A hacker who just noses about an illicitly viewed medical chart, and then forgets all about it, has *wronged* someone – even if that someone never learns of the breach. No harm is done, but powerful moral intuitions tell us that efforts to prevent such wrongs must be as diligent as efforts to prevent harms.

Is the use of personal health information without consent to improve patient safety, say, a wrong? We will address that question and others like it in Chapter 8, on research and electronically stored patient information. To get started here, however, we should introduce Fulana Jones-Smyth, who was born on April 1, 2010, in Peoria, Illinois, United States, weighing 3.5 kilograms, and died on July 10, 2080 in Flitwick, Bedfordshire, United Kingdom. If Fulana's daughter were to argue that public availability of those facts constituted a violation of her mother's confidentiality, we should regard the daughter as having missed an important point about vital statistics. Suppose the daughter further held that the public counters or indexes for birth weight and leukemia deaths (the number of 3.5 kg babies born in Peoria in 2014 increased by 1, and the number of people who died in Bedfordshire in 2080 increased by 1) were also illicit because it was *her mother*, specifically her being born and dying, who, without giving her permission to be counted, increased the numbers. If she maintained *that*, even if no one else knew that or could discover it was Fulana Jones-Smyth, then surely we should regard the daughter as a deranged zealot. Fortunately, no one seriously argues against the collection of vital statistics data, or, if someone did, we should regard them similarly.

Suppose further that under the Transatlantic/International Process for Sustainable Inquiry, established in 2059, data aggregators and analysts determine that World Citizen 7s3j9t5p9r2m5y1z4:

- was born on November 1, 2010, in Peoria, Illinois, United States
- weighed 3.5 kilograms at birth
- had Apgar scores of 2,2,2,2,1
- received usual vaccinations throughout childhood
- broke her arm at the age of 14 in a misadventure involving a horse
- was successfully treated for chlamydia twice between the ages of 20 and 30
- was twice misdiagnosed as having that malady during the same period
- never smoked
- never married
- had one daughter
- worked episodically in ceramic factories
- participated at the age of 31 in a survey about sexual behavior in young women; the aggregate results were published in the *Southern Midwest Journal of Socially Complicated Maladies*
- was tested at a High Street Greengrocer and Genetic Testing Service and found to have a p53 mutation
- had mild osteoporosis
- was hospitalized thrice in her 60s in Britain and the United States for shortness of breath
- ...
- died July 10, 2080 in Flitwick, Bedfordshire, United Kingdom, of adenocarcinoma of the lung

If all that and more information – excepting her name – were available to people working for public health authorities or trusted governance systems, would we say "7s3j9t5p9r2m5y1z4" had been wronged (before or after she died)? Would we really want to suggest that anything learned about lung cancer or improving diagnostic accuracy or the incidence of osteoporosis was wrongly learned?

Perhaps the greatest damage done by lack of confidence in the security of health records is manifested in patient reluctance to tell the full truth about potentially stigmatizing facts. As we saw, it is commonplace for patients to deceive physicians or withhold information about drug use (including alcohol and nicotine), sexual behavior, diet, and the like or for patients to reveal this information but then to ask their doctors not to include it in the medical record. That such stigmatizing information is easily available from an electronic medical record should provide special incentives for clinicians and institutions to adopt robust security measures and strict access policies. Of course, at least some problems of trust and confidentiality will persist unless society decides that people should not be stigmatized or penalized for their illnesses in the first place. In the meantime, and as we will see again in Chapter 8, there is a strong case to be made that while privacy and confidentiality are precious, we esteem other values as well, and some or many of them increase safety, reduce error, improve care, and guide public health. Designed well and used correctly, privacy protections and structures can help us respect those values as well.

Notes

1. The United States: www.hhs.gov/ocr/privacy/ and www.gpo.gov/fdsys/pkg/FR-2013-01-25/pdf/2013-01073. pdf. EU: ec.europa.eu/justice/data-protection/index_en.htm and http://eur-lex.europa.eu/LexUriServ/LexU riServ.do?uri=CELEX:31995L0046:en:HTML. UK: www.legislation.gov.uk/ukpga/1998/29/contents and www.legislation.gov.uk/ukpga/1998/42/contents.

2. Indeed, it could be any clinic and for any malady or purpose. We will visit the issue of HIV/AIDS and other "exceptionalisms" later.

3. Hippocrates, his students, or the Pythagoreans; cf. Chapter 2, note 3; and Chapter 4, note 3.

4. Note omitted. It was 40 years later, in his dissent in *Olmstead* v. *U.S.*, 277 U.S. 438, a prohibition-era case involving the wiretapping of a liquor seller, that Brandeis famously framed the concept of privacy as a "right to be let alone."

5. The world's largest health care data breach apparently occurred in early 2015 when as many as 80 million medical identification numbers – but apparently not medical records – were stolen by hackers who also took Social Security numbers and other data from Anthem, an Indianapolis, Indiana-based insurance company (Abelson and Creswell 2015). In 2011, a National Health Service laptop computer with 8.3 million patient records was stolen; and in 2009 more than 8.2 million records were stolen from Virginia Department of Health Professions servers. See "World's Largest Data Breaches," from David McCandless' "Information Is Beautiful" Web site (www.informationisbeautiful.net/visualizations/worlds-biggest-data-breaches-hacks/.) Note also the "How Much Is Your Hacked Data Worth?" table, which gives the black market price of various data, including "health credentials used to buy drugs or make fake insurance claims," or about $10 in early 2015.

6. Public Law 111–148, available at www.gpo.gov/fdsys/pkg/PLAW-111publ148/html/PLAW-111publ148.htm.

7. Public Law 233, available at www.gpo.gov/fdsys/pkg/PLAW-110publ233/html/PLAW-110publ233.htm.

8. See www.hhs.gov/ocr/privacy/hipaa/understanding/coveredentities/minimumnecessary.html.

9. From the Privacy by Design organization's Web site:

   Privacy by Design advances the view that the future of privacy cannot be assured solely by compliance with legislation and regulatory frameworks; rather, privacy assurance must ideally become an organization's default mode of operation ... Initially, deploying Privacy–Enhancing Technologies (PETs) was seen as the solution. Today, we understand that a more substantial approach is required – extending the use of PETs to taking a positive–sum, not a zero-sum, approach," www.privacybydesign.ca/index.php/about-pbd/applications/.

From the UK Information Commissioner's Office: "Privacy by design is an approach to projects that promotes privacy and data protection compliance from the start. Unfortunately, these issues are often bolted on as an after-thought or ignored altogether … Although this approach is not a requirement of the Data Protection Act, it will help organisations comply with their obligations under the legislation … The ICO encourages organisations to ensure that privacy and data protection is a key consideration in the early stages of any project, and then throughout its lifecycle," https://ico.org.uk/for-organisations/guide-to-data-pro tection/privacy-by-design/.

10. See http://hl7.org/implement/standards/fhir/v3/Confidentiality/ and http://hl7.org/implement/standards/ fhir/v3/Confidentiality/v3-Confidentiality.xml.html.

11. The subsequent HITECH Act strengthened "the regulations that affect the collection, use and disclosure of health information not only by covered entities, but also the 'business associates' (contractors) of those covered entities, and other types of organizations engaged in health information exchange" (Goodman et al. 2014, 349). HITECH, or the Health Information Technology for Economic and Clinical Health Act, was a component of the American Recovery and Reinvestment Act of 2009, or Public Law 111–5, the success of which pulled the United States from the brink of economic disaster during the Great Recession and was one of President Barack Obama's greatest achievements.

12. Available at http://eur-lex.europa.eu/legal-content/en/ALL/?uri=CELEX:31995L0046. Note long-standing contemplation of nontrivial and controversial revisions.

13. Indeed, there is also a scale for measuring "self stigma" (Boyd et al. 2014). The stigma and exceptionalism literature is vast. Some selections: Green and Botkin 2003; Holzemer et al. 2007; Stangl et al. 2013.

14. A very useful overview of some of these issues is to be found in a 1998 US Department of Health and Human Services white paper, "Unique Health Identifier for Individuals" (http://aspe.hhs.gov/admnsimp/nprm/ noiwp1.htm, accessed January 2015), which allows that:

Controversy over the adoption of a standard for the unique health identifier for individuals has focused, to a large degree, on privacy concerns. Some of these views contrast sharply with the previous discussion of the value a unique identifier for individuals would have in clinical practice. We should stress that these privacy issues are substantive, not a trivial concern or a public relations matter. For some, privacy threats outweigh any practical benefits of improved patient care or administrative savings. To others, privacy concerns are significant, but can be managed. To some, the status quo poses greater privacy risks.

15. The report's summary findings (pp. 3–4):
   1. Standardized patient identifying attributes should be required in the relevant exchange transactions.
   2. Any changes to patient data attributes in exchange transactions should be coordinated with organizations working on parallel efforts to standardize healthcare transactions.
   3. Certification criteria should be introduced that require certified EHR technology (CEHRT) to capture the data attributes that would be required in the standardized patient identifying attributes.
   4. The ability of additional, non-traditional data attributes to improve patient matching should be studied.
   5. Certification criteria should not be created for patient matching algorithms or require organizations to utilize a specific type of algorithm.
   6. Certification criteria that requires [sic] CEHRT that performs patient matching to demonstrate the ability to generate and provide to end users reports that detail potential duplicate patient records should be considered.
   7. Build on the initial best practices that emerged during the environmental scan by convening industry stakeholders to consider a more formal structure for establishing best practices for the matching process and data governance.
   8. Work with the industry to develop best practices and policies to encourage consumers to keep their information current and accurate.

9. Work with healthcare professional associations and the Safety Assurance Factors for EHR Resilience (SAFER) Guide initiative to develop and disseminate educational and training materials detailing best practices for accurately capturing and consistently verifying patient data attributes.

10. Continue collaborating with federal agencies and the industry on improving patient identification and matching processes.

Professionalism, programming, and pedagogy

4

Electronic health records are essential for high-quality health care – at least those who advocate their ubiquitous adoption are convinced of this, and not without good reason. But the counterpoint to EHR hosannas is a suite of concerns about the risk of erosion of traditional skills and relationships, new species of unprofessional behaviors, and unintended consequences, including corruption of the traditional – and by some lights sacred – medical record by harried and hurried clinicians copying and pasting dated, and sometimes inaccurate, notes. Moreover, what it means to be a professional in an informatics world now requires attention to the role of information technologies in skill degradation, the responsible conduct of research, and in replicating or corroborating the results of prior research.

Foundations, history, and challenges

A professional once was one who professes, as in one who professes vows or makes a commitment. "Professor" has the same etymology. The term is difficult to use precisely, in part, because it admits of numerous uses. In loose talk, a football player, chef, or prostitute might be a professional for no reason other than being paid, perhaps well, for something others might consider doing without remuneration; perhaps they do it better. More rigorous uses imply the following: A professional is one who has special knowledge or skills, has been credentialed, certified, or licensed, and hews to a special code of conduct or ethics, or takes an oath. But even these criteria might be inadequate to distinguish a profession from an occupation. Generally and minimally, "For most researchers, professions are regarded as essentially the knowledge-based category of service occupations which usually follow a period of tertiary education and vocational training and experience" (Evetts 2013, 781).

Surely, though, some undertakings are uncontroversially those of professionals. As such, listing medicine, nursing, psychology, epidemiology, and pharmacy should not invite dissent. At any rate, these, and researchers in these fields, are primarily the professionals whose behavior we are concerned with. All these professions are served, more or less well, by professional organizations that publish codes of conduct.[1] Some codes are general and are intended to apply to all in the profession; some are developed by specialist societies; overwhelmingly most are geographically limited and apply to a particular province, state, or country (exceptions being a number of international codes for human-subject protection[2]). Medical oaths by students or new physicians are much more common in the United States than in Britain, this being explained by the former's custom of swearing allegiance to a flag (BMJ 2001).

Codes of ethics are tricky to write and to follow. If they are too broad, it is not clear what they require or forbid, and, if they are too specific, it is not clear precisely which actions they permit; it is often recommended that codes be revisited and revised from time to time (Goodman 1996b). Much the same is true of oaths, the best known of which in the health professions is the Hippocratic Oath, the problem with which is that it contains provisions objectionable to many physicians.[3]

The writing of codes of ethics has become a kind of growth industry, driven, it may be hypothesized, by the belief that such a document will guide or improve behavior. It might even be that ethics codes are believed to confer an aura of integrity on institutions otherwise lacking in integrity: The Enron Corp. had a code of ethics, famous now as an exemplar of window dressing to paper over corporate venality, corruption, and sleaze (Sims and Brinkmann 2003). Having employees sign a statement that they have received (and read?) a code, as is custom in some institutions, and as was Enron's policy, seems to be based on the idea that a professional is more likely to hew to a code if she says she received a copy and read it (cf. Chapter 6). That might be true, but it also grates against the idea that a professional is someone we might have hoped would behave in a certain way simply and precisely *because* she is a professional. That is, the concept of "professional" should include the idea that an individual, in part by virtue of training and education, will adhere to standards for no reason other than that one ought to. Put differently, if the threat of punishment is required to guide behavior, then one's development has been arrested at the earliest stage of Kohlbergian moral growth. We should not congratulate a nurse or physician, say, who refrains from having sex with a patient solely out of fear of reprimand or the loss of a license to practice.

To be a professional is in part a stance, the minimum form of commitment, toward standards, best practices, and even custom. Professionalism and ethics can be difficult to disentangle, partly because of the role of tradition and custom. Some actions forbidden by one profession may be permitted in another. It is uncontroversially unprofessional (and in some jurisdictions illegal) for a physician to receive monetary compensation for referring a patient to a colleague; this is sometimes called a "kick-back." In the practice of law, however, many jurisdictions permit "referral fees" for precisely the same purpose.

Health information technology is at the intersection of two vast areas of human inquiry and activity: the health professions and the computing and information technology professions. The former generally require extensive training, often including exposure to issues in professionalism and ethics, and the latter less so; medical training is in part a function of long-standing requirements for the accreditation of medical and nursing schools, and residency programs. But the standards and requirements can be quite recent. ABET (formerly the Accreditation Board for Engineering and Technology, the acronym being preferred to acknowledge the growth of computer science programs) has established ethics and professionalism standards for less than 20 years.

If professionalism entails a stance or commitment, then it remains for the various professions to identify what it is that practitioners should commit to. This articulation of values is a great challenge and, indeed, one of the virtues of attempting to craft a code of ethics in the first place. We often teach medicine and nursing students to care for patients independently of the patients' ability to pay – but does this apply to all patients? Always? Come what may? The *American College of Physicians Ethics Manual* declares that:

The patient–physician relationship entails special obligations for the physician to serve the patient's interest because of the specialized knowledge that physicians possess, the confidential nature of the relationship, and the imbalance of power between patient and physician. Physicians publicly profess that they will use their skills for the benefit of patients, not their own benefit. Physicians must uphold this declaration, as should their professional associations as communities of physicians that put patient welfare first.[4]

While many physicians adopt this stance, many also do not. Are they behaving unprofessionally? If so, what, if anything, is to be done? Must engineers and computer scientists demonstrate "an ability to communicate effectively," per ABET standards[5] – really? Always? The Association for Computing Machinery's "Code of Ethics and Professional Conduct" begins "*As an ACM member I will* ... Contribute to society and human well-being."[6] This is as vague as it is noble, and a seemingly very high bar to meet.

The field of health informatics is inhabited by physicians, nurses, dentists, and biomedical researchers, as well as by computer scientists, computer programmers, electronic communications specialists, and systems analysts and designers. Such diversity notwithstanding, the American Board of Medical Specialties established in 2013 a new certification in clinical informatics; that is, one can now be board certified in clinical informatics. Championed by AMIA (formerly the American Medical Informatics Association), such certification adds an additional threshold to the house of professional education and standards.

The challenge of crafting a code for this new profession is shaped in part by the fact that if one is a nurse, for instance, or a computer scientist, say, one is already engaged in an activity with several applicable codes. What is special or unique about health informatics? Should an informatician attend to confidentiality issues more than a psychologist or pharmacist who lives a computer-free life? Does the diverse practice of informatics require a commitment to patient-centeredness at least as strong as (or no stronger than that of) a physician? The informatics community is served by two professional organizations, AMIA and the International Medical Informatics Association, both of which have grappled with and delivered codes of ethics. In the case of AMIA, the questions just posed loomed large and were subject to extensive debate. The resulting code is brief – a 1-page introduction and a 1-page set of guiding "principles," for instance:

> Members of the Ethics Committee are unanimous in the view that those who work in informatics – much as in other health professions – are duty-bound to embrace a patient-centered approach to their work, even if that work does not involve direct patient care or human subjects research. As elsewhere in the health professions, vulnerable populations or those with special needs may be entitled to additional considerations.
>
> (Goodman et al. 2013, 141)

While the invocation of "patient-centered care" is pedestrian, the notion that even non-clinicians should embrace it is not. Such a requirement emerged after debate about the code's force and scope, and the extent to which hewing to it would be the mark of a professional. The code also counsels that AMIA members "Not mislead patients about the collection, use, or communication of their healthcare information" (ibid., 142). Now compare similar duties enumerated by the IMIA code:

> [Health Informatics Professionals] have a duty to ensure that the subject of an electronic record is made aware that

a. an electronic record has been established about her/him,
b. who has established the record and who continues to maintain it,
c. what is contained in the electronic record,
d. the purpose for which it is established,
e. the individuals, institutions or agencies who have access to it or to whom it (or an identifiable part of it) may be communicated,
f. where the electronic record is maintained,
g. the length of time it will be maintained, and
h. the ultimate nature of its disposition.[7]

The former is brief, even telegraphic, to the point that it is not clear what a professional's duties are under the code. The latter is detailed – so much so that it is possible to worry that no one has ever adhered to it. This underscores anew the difficulties encountered in trying to draft codes of ethics or conduct.

A desirable feature of codes is that they should not be controversial; that is, they should not themselves engender (much) debate. Whether lofty or quotidian, a document intended to inform and guide the behavior of professionals should capture what is settled or agreed to in the profession. When practice varies, or varies widely, it is a signal that what is the case and what ought to be the case are not in alignment. Only a change in the profession's culture or standards can resolve this disjunction. Now, it might be the case that a code should strive to be aspirational – but even here there will be a tension between the code-writer's vision and the practice of her adherents. In all cases and as above, it is probably wise to counsel that a code be reassessed and revised every so often. The AMIA code, for instance, first appeared in 2007 and was revised in 2011 – after which the organization's Ethics Committee immediately set about preparing for the next version.

Perhaps what is wanted in a discussion of professionalism in health information technology, where it has been suggested that the technology requires "a new version of the physician-patient relationship with respect to health information" (Rothstein 2010, 11),[8] are analyses of those issues and practices that are emerging, perhaps novel, yet important, or that are so large they do not initially appear to be salient for some or many of those in the profession. Our task in what follows will be to do just that, namely, analyze professionalism challenges related to skill degradation, copying and pasting in the electronic health record, the responsible conduct of research, and the replication and reproducibility of scientific results. The last two of these are a source of intense contemporary debate – vast deliberations that bear on nothing less than the success of modern health care. Significantly, for our purposes, they require the use of health information technology.

Skill degradation

Every generation enjoys the services of at least a few pessimists who despair of the current state of affairs, or the direction in which things are going. It is good sport, even if it is difficult to tell who is winning. The growing use of computers and information technology in the health professions has been a rich source of speculation concerning its effect on the traditional skills of clinicians. These are among the questions that concern us:

1. Do computers cause skill degradation or improve clinical skills?
2. Do computers "deprofessionalize" clinicians?
3. Do computers improve or impede the clinician–patient relationship?

Concerns that health information technology might cause or is already causing a reduction in clinicians' skill set require an itemization of the skills at issue. In the broadest sense, the practice of medicine or nursing is profoundly human: One asks intimate questions of another, observes another, and touches another; palpates, perhaps painfully, gives powerful medicines, and rends skin; communicates about illness, disability, and death. Managing this relationship with compassion and equanimity is one of the marks of a professional. Any machine that improves human ability to do these things is probably a good machine. But it might not be a good thing if the machine merely makes it easier for the clinician. Making something easier for one does not necessarily make it better for the other.

In Chapter 1 we looked at contradictory evidence regarding the use and utility of electronic health records. We saw, recall, that the arrival of electronic health records can be likened to a "third party" in the exam room, or one "that reshapes the patient-physician encounter, alters the patient's narrative, and diverts the physician's attention away from the patient. This diminishes the patient-centeredness of interactions, which in turn affects the patient-physician relationship" (Lown and Rodriguez 2012, 392).

Overarchingly, the fear that might be worth having is that computers and their medical accessories cause or risk damage to the human element in health care (Shortliffe 1993, 1994), perhaps by eroding specific skills. This is a difficult empirical question, especially when framed broadly, as here. There is a growing literature on this topic, albeit generally about individuals' "satisfaction" with new technology, and sometimes about impediments and improvements to communication – something clinicians have a poor-to-mediocre record of in the first place, especially when the stakes are high (Penson et al. 2006). (That is to say, most anything to improve end-of-life communication is likely to be welcomed.) For that matter, what if this cherished "human element" were diminished – but patients were cured sooner, suffered less, and lived longer? If so, what then was the basis for our fear? Edward H. Shortliffe, a pioneer in and key contributor to the field of biomedical informatics, is likely right, though it will yet be some time before most agree:

> the mere existence of computers as tools for physicians and other health workers need not be a threat to our goal of humane care, with close relationships developing between patients and caregivers … As computers recede into the environment, but increasingly help physicians find information quickly and easily, the result may be a release of time that will become available for building precisely the kind of caring relationships that both patients and physicians have always sought. (Shortliffe 1993, 397)

Indeed, there is a dearth of empirical studies documenting the effect of health information technology on actual clinical skills. Rather, there are reports of physicians and others saying they have lost, or fear they are losing, skills (e.g., Friedberg et al. 2013; Harris 1990). But precisely what skills are clinicians afraid of losing?[9]

It might be communications skills, but if these are poor to begin with, we will not have a useful baseline against which to measure change. Indeed, it has been suggested that making patients partners in medical documentation might help in *improving* this valuable skill (Walker et al. 2011); or, independently of whether it improves any particular skill, it might simply result in better documentation. It has also been suggested, with some evidentiary support, that the use of medical scribes can decouple physicians from their computers – freeing them for direct patient care and direct communication – and improve the quality of medical documentation (Bastani et al. 2014; Brady and Shariff 2013; Gellert et al. 2014). To be sure, the use of scribes introduces a human "third party," the effects of which remain an interesting topic for future research.

Perhaps, then, the use of decision support systems can be shown to degrade diagnostic skills. One physician in Texas blames templates in his electronic health record for "trying its hardest every day to make me worse" at being a doctor and rendering accurate diagnoses (Urban 2010). A complicated study would be required to determine if this is an actual and widespread phenomenon. Indeed, one might hypothesize that the use of decision support systems, especially their ability to identify and rank differential diagnoses, might actually improve diagnostic acumen. Remember, we are not here assessing whether decision support systems can help render diagnoses more accurately or not, or otherwise improve care, or not (cf. Berner et al. 1999) – rather, we are looking for evidence in support of the conjecture that a human skill has itself been, or will be, diminished.

Maybe we should inquire whether health information technology decreases skills generally, so that without such technology a clinician is less able to practice competently. This would be akin to learning phlebotomy or suturing in school but then losing the ability to do either after a period of time in a practice requiring neither. Is there any evidence for this in informatics? One may sympathize with the intuition at work here: Surely dependence on a machine will cause a reduction in an ability that predated the dependence. But even if this is the case for something like auscultation, say – use of a stethoscope might degrade the ability to auscultate without one – it is the use of a tool that uncontroversially improves care such that wistfulness about the old skill ought not be dignified by the sentiment.[10] In addition, we do sometimes mourn the fact that students and residents order too many laboratory tests or imaging studies, but our concern here is shaped by the knowledge that such tests and studies are often unnecessary and unnecessarily costly. It is not that the trainees have lost a skill – it is at least as likely that they never acquired it in the first place.

What about education? Might it be that health information technology, including simulators and computer-controlled manikins, when used in training and education, produces less-competent clinicians? In fact, the evidence shows quite the opposite. Health pedagogy technologies are good for trainees, can reduce error, and fledge and improve skills (BMJ 2009; Cook et al. 2011; Reynolds and Kong 2011; Treloar et al. 2001; Ward and Wattier 2011).

While the risk of skill degradation caused (or permitted) by health information technology is not implausible, it is a complex and rich empirical question about which there is precious little data. To the extent that a professional or intellectual community can have a collective moral obligation, this community should strive to gather more data. Individual clinicians should be attentive and committed, as one should assume they were always were, to maintaining and, indeed, improving their skills.

CTRL-A, CTRL-C, CTRL-V: the challenge of copying and pasting in the electronic health record

The human inclination to identify means of reducing or simplifying labor is a sensible curiosity. It is sensible because some or much work is boring. It is or can be a curiosity because not all reductions or simplifications increase efficiency or productivity, which is evolutionarily counterproductive. In any case, one evolving contemporary practice is a good candidate as an exemplar of the deprofessionalization of clinical practice.

The temptation to copy and paste elements of yesterday's hospital problem list, for instance, from the medical record is apparently a temptation not only too difficult to resist but also apparently increasingly widespread (issues addressed in this section are variably introduced by the following: Hartzband and Groopman 2008; Hirschtick 2006; Siegler 2010; Siegler and Adelman 2009; Thielke et al. 2007; Weis and Levy 2014).

If copying and pasting were merely transposing yesterday's facts accurately to today's note – that is, if one were to confirm that yesterday's facts are still today's – then it would still lead to a disruptive and confusing bloating of a document whose uses include helping and guiding other caregivers. That is, copying and pasting might be a means of bringing information forward, but it is also driven in part by the need for documentation for the sake of billing, at least in some jurisdictions; a detailed list provides undergirding for the time spent with a patient, even if it does not advance the care of the patient. If information, even accurate information, is merely repeated, it is of comparatively little use in helping to shape that care; it might even make such care more difficult if salient details are not highlighted or if changes are not made explicit. In some cases, copying and pasting has led to extraordinary bloating of the record.

Worse, the accuracy just assumed is too often not the case. A mistake copied becomes a mistake repeated, if not immortalized. As a note in the record increases in detail and as it is copied more frequently, the greater the difficulty in identifying errors. In hospitals that (continue to) maintain an isomorphic paper record, conflicts between the electronic and paper records can pose great impediments to the care of patients. One can imagine a three- or even an n-way conflict among elements in the chart. This is especially a problem at hospitals, such as at academic medical centers, with many trainees and frequent turnover of attending physicians. When the stakes are high, the consequences can be dramatic. Imagine copying a note for a patient with a do-not-resuscitate order after the DNR has been rescinded, or vice versa.

Another problem with copying and pasting is the risk of a loss of authorship, or of the origin or provenance of an observation or a measurement. If it is true that communication between and among clinicians is an essential component of high-quality care, then identifying the source of a particular finding is important. The only way to be sure that one has the right source is to have carefully reviewed previous notes in an effort to find the point at which a datum was introduced or changed. While this is not impossible, it can turn a busy clinician into a kind of detective engaged in the time-wasting and stupefying task of text analysis. Copying and pasting can waste colleagues' time and, in itself and in consequence, can impede patient care.

It is not wholly clear if copying and pasting deprofessionalizes clinicians or if those already deprofessionalized are more likely to seek its succor. Clinicians should be forgiven, at least a little. If we have learned anything from the study of medical error, it is that overwhelmingly most errors follow a sequence of events in which one or more underpinned the error. That is to say, medical errors are often the result of a failure of a system imposed on or adopted by institutions. This is certainly true of many, if not most, electronic health records. This is because the original commercial electronic health records in use in most hospitals and practices were not designed or developed foremostly to maximize the use of information technology to improve patient care. As it became clear that documentation on paper was an inadequate way of communicating patient information, it was also realized that electronic records could produce a detailed and documented history to support billing and reimbursement. Moreover, many electronic health records are, as we have seen, difficult to use: They are organized in such a way that they seem to pay little attention to the information that the clinician or patient needs and are uncooperative in producing important information easily.

None of this is the fault of doctors or nurses on whom inferior products have been imposed. Although they must to some extent play with the cards they've been dealt, this does not absolve them, or others, from the duty to advocate for better systems. Many institutions have created teams of informatics champions to work to improve systems, though that, too, poses challenges. One could disable the copy-and-paste function, though that risks turning clever trainees into hackers, where a better course might be to:

> change the nature of the house staff progress note. Admission histories and physical examinations would remain the same, comprehensive and complete. To document progress, however, interns could write a *brief* narrative, describing the events and plans for the day. Residents could write a structured note on a core of patients, with the explicit goal of learning how to document accurately and how to bill correctly. Attendings, in exchange for strong house staff notes to which they can link, could spend more time clarifying or amplifying and less time in duplicative efforts. The chart would reflect the differing perspectives of all its physician contributors, and the notes might add up to a more complete and more satisfying whole.
> (Siegler and Adelman 2009, 496, original emphasis; cf. AHIMA 2009)

Copying and pasting is not always malign. It does not always constitute evidence of laziness. Limited copying can improve accuracy, and one should not avoid quotation to stand on the ceremony of not copying and pasting if such copying can both save time and maintain accuracy. In such instances, however, one should use quotation marks and include the date and perhaps the author of the material being copied.[11]

In all cases, the mark of a professional in these contexts will be whether one is mindful of and attends to the needs of others. If the practice is solely for the convenience of the copier-paster, then, given the risks to patients and waste of colleagues' time, it is a mark of unprofessionalism and, indeed, might be unethical. This issue, and institutions' response to it, is another example of the potential utility of an appropriately educated hospital ethics committee.

Informatics and the responsible conduct of research

We have for more than a generation witnessed a global upwelling of interest in what is now formally known as the "responsible conduct of research" (RCR). Inspired, or perhaps, better, elicited, by a number of public and noteworthy cases of biomedical scientists who had been found, or were at least suspected of, mishandling research data, RCR initiatives have flourished at professional organizations and academic and other research institutions. In some countries, academic institutions have adopted RCR programs at least in part because of government mandate.

In the United States, for instance, the National Institutes of Health began in 1989 to call for RCR education for all grantees and, as of 2011, requires "all trainees, fellows, participants, and scholars receiving support through any NIH training, career development award (individual or institutional), research education grant, and dissertation research grant must receive instruction in responsible conduct of research."[12] Grant applicants are required to provide details of their RCR education program, and, therefore:

> NIH policy requires participation in and successful completion of instruction in responsible conduct of research by individuals supported by any NIH training/research education/ fellowship/career award. It is expected that course attendance is monitored and that a certificate or documentation of participation is available upon course completion. NIH does not require certification of compliance or submission of documentation, but expects institutions to maintain records sufficient to demonstrate that NIH-supported trainees, fellows, and scholars have received the required instruction.

Also in 2011, Canada's Panel on Responsible Conduct of Research published the "Tri-Agency Framework: Responsible Conduct of Research,"[13] with a section on "Promoting Awareness and Education," specifically:

> a. An Institution is responsible for:
> b. Promoting awareness of what constitutes the responsible conduct of research, including Agency requirements as set out in the Institution's policies, the consequences of failing to meet them, as well as the process for addressing allegations, to all those engaged in research activities at the Institution.
> c. Communicating its policy on the responsible conduct of research within the Institution, and making public statistical annual reports on confirmed findings of breaches of that policy and actions taken, subject to applicable laws, including the privacy laws.
> d. Communicating within the Institution, the central point of contact responsible for receiving confidential enquiries, allegations and information related to allegations of breaches of Agency policies.

The British "Concordat to Support Research Integrity," developed by a consortium of funding agencies, universities, and the Wellcome Trust, committed in 2012 to:

> Maintaining the highest standards in research requires the right environment. It is the responsibility of employers of researchers – and all those undertaking, supporting or otherwise engaged with research – to maintain a culture that nurtures good practice. This includes universities, research institutes, funders of research, professional and representative bodies, and organisations with a regulatory role. ... A research environment that helps to develop good research practice and embeds a culture of research integrity should, as a minimum, include:
> • clear policies, practices and procedures to support researchers
> • suitable learning, training and mentoring opportunities to support the development of researchers ...[14]

A report from the European Commission tries to capture the scope of the challenge:

> Indeed, the scientific community's attempt to regulate itself through the eradication of fabrication, falsification, and plagiarism, to examine questionable research practices such as data manipulation and multiple publication, and to pursue the responsible conduct of research are to be commended and deserve support from the larger society. But the discussions of [fabrication, falsification, and plagiarism, questionable research practices] and RCR also opens up a space for a broader and more substantive consideration of what counts as good or valuable science. Under pressure from national governments and private

corporations to deliver economic growth, science has been asked to redefine its own sense
of integrity and to become self-critical of its social contexts. This is a valuable exercise,
nevertheless limited by national borders and a tendency to remain within narrow bounds.
(Ozoliņa et al. 2009, 27; cf. European Science Foundation 2011)

While laboratory science is mistakenly not often thought of as a profession in the same way
as its clinical cousins, certainly the world's biomedical and other scientists comprise a
profession, and, equally surely, most laboratory scientists view themselves as having to
note, mark, attend to, or comply with standards of precisely the sort that apply to and
govern other professions. Moreover, and especially for our purposes, the role of informatics
in laboratory science is too often unrecognized and therefore neglected. The goal here is to
make laboratory scientists full partners in the ethics-and-informatics ambit.

Consider that while no formal curriculum is required or specified, the NIH identifies
nine topics as having "been incorporated into most acceptable plans for such instruction":[15]

a. conflict of interest – personal, professional, and financial
b. policies regarding human subjects, live vertebrate animal subjects in research, and safe
   laboratory practices
c. mentor/mentee responsibilities and relationships
d. collaborative research including collaborations with industry[16]
e. peer review
f. data acquisition and laboratory tools; management, sharing, and ownership
g. research misconduct and policies for handling misconduct
h. responsible authorship and publication
i. the scientist as a responsible member of society, contemporary ethical issues in
   biomedical research, and the environmental and societal impacts of scientific research

Each of these topics can be seen to lend itself to an assessment of issues at the seam between
ethics and computing – trivially, in that all of them make use of information technology to
some extent or another, and, substantially, in that data acquisition, management, and
sharing, and, nowadays, publication and authorship, are explicitly computational. This is
also where the most visible scientific misconduct occurs; that is, fabrication, falsification,
and plagiarism have become cyber-wrongs in the twenty-first century.

The modern laboratory is intensely computational, with scientists writing, borrowing,
and modifying software as an essential component of their work.[17] A survey by Britain's
Software Sustainability Institute found that 92% of academic scientists use research software, 69% reported their research "would not be practical without it," 56% said they develop
their own software (of whom 21% have no training in software development), and 70% of
males and 30% of females develop their own software (Hettrick 2014). More than 40% of
those surveyed used Python, R, or SPSS, all familiar in biomedical or social science labs.

This is a fertile plain. Scientists have evolved into programmers in the past half-century,
and this has changed the feel and fabric of the modern laboratory. The tools of the modern
lab are also run by computers. Gene sequencers, microarrays, and even balances are digital.
They are fed a piece of the world, and render it machine-readable. Laboratory science has
become computational.

Some inappropriate uses of computers in biomedical laboratory science are pedestrian.
The NIH Office of Research Integrity regularly publishes "Findings of Research
Misconduct," documenting instances of fabrication and falsification mediated by

information technology and found in grant applications and publications of the results of research funded by the government. An increasingly common stratagem is the use of photo-manipulation software to alter images, often of western blot or microarray images to create the impression of a lab finding not made or a result that did not occur. One might use basic computer tools to fabricate or falsify data to produce a factitious result. Consider an Office of Research Integrity account of a researcher sanctioned in 2014. The government reported that the investigator:

> created a hierarchy of computer folders containing duplicated and renamed files; the falsified groups of files included eighty-two (82) groups of duplicated files with each group containing two to twenty-one (2–21) duplicates, which made it appear that experiments were conducted when they were not used the falsified and/or fabricated data files in Figure 6 of a paper published ... to represent Ca+ currents in cardiac myocytes from CLCAD-/- mice; specifically, Respondent claimed that Figure 6 represented results from seven (7) mice when the data files were three (3) sets of duplicated and renamed files plus one additional data file. All of the data files were part of larger groups of identical duplicated and renamed data files on the Respondent's hard drive.

Examples like this are not particularly interesting. That they exemplify wrongdoing is not in dispute. It is not even clear that the use of information technology is essential to the wrongdoing – one might retouch a photo by traditional means or mislabel a paper file folder with a pencil to (try to) achieve the same effect as intentionally mislabeling a digital file. It might be that the availability of computer tools makes such temptations more difficult to resist or detect, but that is not our concern here, any more than the fact that automobiles are better than horse-drawn carriages to enable a getaway after a bank robbery is not essential to the understanding that one ought not to rob banks.

For the RCR curriculum to include information technology in a nontrivial way, we must look to the history of ethics in software development and computing.

The last quarter-century of the ethics-and-computing literature makes clear that *trust*, the value, is perhaps the most important among all values. Trust, as we will see in Chapter 6, is a product of transparency, veracity, and accountability. Indeed, it underpins empirical beliefs and knowledge (Hardwig 1991) as well as social interactions. Trust is an adhesive that holds civil society together (Hosking 2014). Trust would not be necessary if each individual could verify the truth, quality, or provenance of all the information, products, or services we use. But no one can do that, at least not easily: If one knows enough physics, one can believe in the existence of Higgs bosons without having to rely on others; if I learned enough about automobiles, I could acquire a true belief about the quality of a car I intend to buy; if you learned enough computer programming, and had the time or inclination to check and test a programmer's code in all possible or likely contexts, you would be confident that the program will function as intended. With very rare exceptions, however, most people believe in the existence of Higgs bosons, buy a car, or use software without any such skill or knowledge at all. This is in part because we tend to trust physicists, car sellers, and programmers. Such trust is sometimes, perhaps often, supported by the most slender of threads.

Professor Deborah G. Johnson in her classic *Computer Ethics* (2009; cf. the several valuable contributions in Collste 2000) distinguishes among four relationships shaping the work of computer professionals: employer–employee, client–professional, society–professional, and professional–professional. The last two are most applicable to the purpose here.

A variety of mutual responsibilities arises in the relationship between society and scientist. Society wants more and better biomedical research and so should pay adequately for it and protect it. Equally, the code-writing scientist is duty-bound to deliver the goods, and these products must be of adequate quality; this means that the research that relies on the code written by laboratory workers must meet the standards that maximize, or are believed to maximize, discovery and other goals. We can regard this as quite broad, and then it becomes difficult and perhaps unnecessary to itemize the many other obligations that many people have to society. Therefore, by writing code that is sloppy, undocumented, or overstated, for instance, one has cheated society. This is the case when others rely on the code even if the programmer is not paid by those others.

It is in the professional–professional relationship that these maladaptive software properties or traits emerge as motivating and guiding the content of an RCR curriculum for lab scientists.

Consider the design of a user interface. In 2001, Don Gotterbarn created a scenario in which one Joanne Buildscreen, a software engineer, designed a user interface under government contract that met a manager's specifications and requirements, but was "so hard to use that the complaints ... were heard by ... upper level management" and this led to a halt in development funds, ill-will toward the company, a burden to taxpayers, and reluctance to innovate in the future (Gotterbarn 2001, 222–3). A decade and a half later, a team of researchers from four institutions studied a set of 100 reports of electronic health record safety problems and found that 94% of safety concerns involved "unmet data-display needs in the EHR (i.e., displayed information available to the end user failed to reduce uncertainty or led to increased potential for patient harm), software upgrades or modifications, data transmission between components of the EHR, or 'hidden dependencies' within the EHR" (Meeks et al. 2014; cf. Middleton et al. 2013). While the uninitiated might puzzle over the significance of a user interface, the way it is used to retrieve, represent, and receive information for storage or transmission to others can be a life-and-death matter. It would be interesting to learn how many laboratory mistakes are made and perpetuated by balky user interfaces. Evidence of harms caused by poor interfaces has accelerated the growth of User Centered Design, which takes the bold step of actually having system users participate in system design (Horsky et al. 2012).

In what follows I propose a suite of laboratory programmer duties, all of which fall under the headings transparency, veracity, and accountability/responsibility (again, see Chapter 6 for additional discussion). Each is uncontroversial, and all could easily be included in any RCR program. There are doubtless others worth including. In context, each might require a judgment about the force of terms like "appropriate," "sufficient," and so on. This is among the values of applied ethics: While it should make clear why frank wrongdoing is wrong, it should also guide and inform discussion about cases that might not be obvious. In what follows, the frank wrongdoing would be intentionally to avoid any of the duties. Note that additional values – trust and reliability here, for instance – emerge naturally from acceptance of the others, a kind of moral harmonic supervening on those others.

Write code appropriate to the purpose. While reusing code can be a convenience and a virtue, do not use code developed for one purpose for a different one if the needs of the second purpose are sufficiently different. That is, recycle code only when appropriate. It is more or less appropriate according as it will accomplish the intended task.

Annotate and document carefully. One of the most common laboratory complaints about a colleague's software is how poorly it is annotated and documented. Why is this list here? What does this track do? How does this annotation relate to previous ones? Note in this regard the evolution of collaborative annotation tools. Collaborative annotation, well known in the humanities, where, for instance, a group of students might comment on a text, lies at the juncture of team science and laboratory software engineering.

Identify provenance. Worth a separate item in this list, information about the origin or source of any script, routine, program, and so on is essential to the documentation process. Answering the question, "Where did this come from?" is necessary for intellectual credit and responsibility, as well as to manage circumstances in which a query is required.

Take responsibility as and when appropriate. While collaboration and cooperation generally improve performance, they do not absolve individuals from responsibility for their contribution. A professional is willing to take responsibility. As we saw in Chapter 2, the "problem of many hands" not only can increase complexity of some aspects of software design and application; it similarly can complicate the task of attribution and the assignment of responsibility. This underscores the importance of documenting provenance.

Attend carefully to version control. Anyone who has overwritten a file in error or stared numbly at a screen with two or more versions of the same document will appreciate the importance of version control as an important scientific, social, and ethical issue. Version control is an ethical issue because conflicting or lost versions can waste others' time and institutional resources and impede quality.

So far we have been concerned with the responsible conduct of research curriculum with a comparatively narrow focus. In this section we broaden the focus to include the overarching social responsibilities of programmers in biomedical laboratories. In the same way we might ask graduate students to discuss ethical issues raised by works on nuclear fission, weaponized anthrax, or genetic modification of human traits, say, we might also direct their thoughts to the larger context of their own work. This idea has rarely been better expressed than by Langdon Winner:

> It is obvious that technologies can be used in ways that enhance the power, authority, and privilege of some over others, for example, the use of television to sell a candidate. In our accustomed way of thinking technologies are seen as neutral tools that can be used well or poorly, for good, evil, or something in between. But we usually do not stop to inquire whether a given device might have been designed and built in such a way that it produces a set of consequences logically and temporally *prior to any of its professed uses.*
>
> (1980, 125, original emphasis; cited by Nissenbaum 2000)

There is another way of putting this. It is that professionals cannot escape all social responsibility, at least in some measure. It is no longer (if it has ever been) permissible to declaim that "My work is apolitical, a-ethical and a-social. The purity of my science is a mark of my agnosticism as regards the larger questions and challenges faced by society." Such a stance constitutes an appeal to ignorance and amounts to a surrender to some of the darker forces of academic and corporate inquiry.

Reproducibility, corroboration, and replication of scientific results

A strong case could be made to support the notion that the most compelling reason to introduce software development into the RCR curriculum is the positive effect this could have on scientific reproducibility. This is a kind of pedagogic hypothesis: Information technology is used to analyze and shape laboratory practice and the publications that result from it. Variations in training and practice of those who use this technology are reckoned to contribute to the reproducibility problem. No ill intent is needed for this unfortunate contribution, but if there is anything correct about this hypothesis it could help explain and address the problem.

The growth of laboratory science in the nineteenth and twentieth centuries was driven by many familiar and well-noted forces: curiosity, priority, and fame, and the hope that lab diligence might improve the lot of humans. These motivations were perfectly adequate to drive scientific progress in the days before there was great wealth to be acquired from laboratory toil or genius.[18] They still are, despite the sad opinion, of comparatively recent vintage, that the first, best, or most powerful motivator of scientists is the hope for personal wealth. For most of the history of science, that was simply false.[19]

In any event, the second decade of the twenty-first century is experiencing a kind of crisis of confidence in the ability of science, especially bioscience, to produce accurate and dependable results. The stakes are quite high, and this makes replication and, more importantly, corroboration, an ethical issue.[20] If there is something wrong with the way we do science, the way it is paid for, or the way it is communicated, the results can erode health and well-being, squander tax money, and waste others' time. This is true of laboratory science and, perhaps more so, of clinical research. There are many causes for the failure of reproducibility: cultural mechanisms, including quests for status, promotion, and profit; methodological sloppiness, including faulty statistics, lack of blinding, cell-line misidentification or mismanagement, and inadequately described ingredients or populations; and overhasty, exaggerated, or nontransparent publication, underpublication, and publication bias (Collins and Tabak 2014; Ioannidis 2005, 2014; Lorsch et al. 2014); perhaps even garden-variety greed for intellectual property and frank misconduct contribute. It might even be in part that the world is more complicated than we would like for our ambitions, careers, and sense of scientific self-worth. While all these causes of reproducibility failure have ethical implications, they alone are not the concern here.

Rather, at all points on the bioresearch spectrum – that is, from laboratory bench to animal studies to clinical trials in humans to postmarketing surveillance – someone is using a computer to collect, analyze, and/or transmit data and information; many are writing the computers' programs. This is the concern, and an opportunity.

As mulled earlier, there is nothing ethically interesting about intentionally deceiving colleagues or society about scientific results. Instead, we should be more interested in the consequences of varying standards in software engineering education and practice (see Kush and Goldman 2014; Lau 2009, 2014). If varying standards for the duties itemized in the previous section – software appropriateness, annotation, and documentation, the identification of provenance, responsibility and accountability, and version control – can individually or collectively impede replication and reproducibility, then this variation acquires ethical significance.

In addition to having the soil well tilled by ubiquitous RCR programs, the idea of harmonizing software engineering skills for scientists enjoys creative instantiation in the work of Software Carpentry, a volunteer, transatlantic organization that runs workshops at universities and other institutions.[21] Curriculum components to be embedded in the nine NIH core topics could include discussion of the standards already itemized, as well as issues in data sharing, trust, safety, and quality. Perhaps the greatest task of mentors in the professions is imbuing learners with the values of the profession. It is therefore important to assign competent faculty to the task, lest students be encouraged in the kind of facile "there is no right answer" relativism, which we saw in Chapter 1 is too often mistaken for tolerance or respect for alternative viewpoints. Fabrication, falsification, and plagiarism are not interesting local customs, as neither are writing sloppy, undocumented code, ignoring version control, or overstating a program's functionality. When a difficult judgment is required, as in setting parameters in statistical analysis, the skills of critical thinking are demanded.

Reproducibility and complexity

As the world's scientific community is in a kerfuffle over reproducibility, it would be a shame not to signal the value of including at least a little epistemology in the education of graduate students. For instance, the philosophy of confirmation has long struggled with the problem of what kind, level, or degree of experiment or test is adequate to justify a belief or confirm or verify a hypothesis. It does not matter for the purposes here whether one is a hypothetico-deductivist, say, or a Bayesian, for instance. What matters is the fledging of scientists who care about, and are thoughtful as regards, evidence. It might just be that replication and reproducibility are so challenging because some phenomena are less tractable than we hoped. Moreover, even if we eliminated or resolved the social causes of reproducibility failure, some science will remain challenging and some experiments will be difficult to replicate because it is difficult to control for significant and complex experimental variables. It also might be the case that a line of inquiry is on target but the phenomenon in question is more delicate or intricate than hoped or expected. These are circumstances that call for more science, not necessarily more virtue.

That said, science and ethics are intertwined in the lab. Whether one is a Popperian or not, there is a lesson to be learned from Popper's idea that the more difficult the experimental challenge, the greater the warrant for consequent belief (e.g., Popper 1959/1980). Indeed, some things can be known more or less easily, but a laboratory scientist will do well to be mindful and suspicious of conclusions or results that are too easily or quickly celebrated. Even a "methodological anarchist" in the spirit of Paul Feyerabend (1975/ 1984) can be catholic about methods but not about inferences drawn from them. Perhaps the greatest unnoticed or unremarked conflict of interest of all is the interest an ambitious student has in finding something novel. Computer programming that eases discovery is either very, very good ... or too good to be true. If software is being used, even unintentionally, to paper over cracks in the epistemic firmament, then something unfortunate is happening.

This is an important lesson for translational bioscience. While "bench-to-bedside" research captures important intuitions about the need to conceptualize some bioscience inquiry holistically instead of discretely or episodically,[22] it is vital that a critical or questioning attitude be retained in the search for and publication of results.

Quality if not excellence, accuracy if not precision, verisimilitude if not truth are candidates to be the overarching empirical goals of any laboratory. We might think of them as professional goals, which are different from epistemological goals, methodological goals, social goals, and economic goals. Reaching these goals will require, in varying degrees, the following:

- better education of scientists
- incorporating the epistemology of confirmation
- identifying and exploiting the intersection of ethics and information technology as a resource for educators and scientists

Data management was once a comparatively straightforward matter of writing things down. The logics of confirmation were able to guide a period of great scientific fertility and discovery. If the results of an experiment on Day 2 matched those of Day 1, the process was inferred to have taught us something about the world. But we do not much write notes on paper anymore, and our data are not seen as much as computed. The world is often somewhat more complicated than we wished. The contention here has been that the goals of the responsible conduct of research need to be achieved not only to ensure integrity and foster trust but also to increase the chances of getting it right.

Notes

1. The Illinois Institute of Technology's Online Ethics Codes Project, with support from the US National Science Foundation, lists more than 1,000 ethics codes at http://ethics.iit.edu/ecodes/.

2. The best known are the World Medical Association's "Declaration of Helsinki," available at www.wma.net/en/30publications/10policies/b3/index.html; and the Council for International Organizations of Medical Sciences' "CIOMS International Ethical Guidelines for Biomedical Research Involving Human Subjects," which, along with related documents, is available at www.cioms.ch/index.php/texts-of-guidelines.

3. This famous oath, likely *not* the work of a historical individual, i.e., Hippocrates (cf. Chapter 2, note 1, and Chapter 3, note 2), is rarely if ever sworn as written. For one thing, it is in ancient Greek. More substantially, it is an oath to several gods, beginning "I swear by Apollo the physician, and Aesculapius the surgeon, likewise Hygeia and Panacea, and call all the gods and goddesses to witness, that I will observe and keep this underwritten oath, to the utmost of my power and judgment." Thus, unless one is an Apollonian, that bit must be omitted or altered. Moreover, the code forbids abortion and assisted suicide or active euthanasia. Most contemporary medical students draft their own oaths, drawing from that of Hippocrates, Maimonides, and others. Nowadays, when one tries to make an argument by saying a physician has uttered the Hippocratic Oath and therefore must or must not do something, he is likely mistaken. (Neither does the code include the injunction "first, do no harm.") See Orr et al. (1997).

4. "ACP Ethics Manual Sixth Edition," American College of Physicians 2012, notes omitted, www.acponline.org/running_practice/ethics/manual/manual6th.htm#ref-10. Cf. Snyder 2012.

5. "ABET's Engineering Criteria 2000 and Engineering Ethics: Where Do We Go from Here?" Online Ethics Center for Engineering, June 26, 2006, National Academy of Engineering, www.onlineethics.org/Education/instructessays/herkert2.aspx.

6. "ACM Code of Ethics and Professional Conduct," October 1992, www.acm.org/about/code-of-ethics.

7. "The IMIA Code of Ethics for Health Information Professionals," October 4, 2001, www.imia-medinfo.org/new2/pubdocs/Ethics_Eng.pdf.

8. See also Goldstein (2010) for a useful discussion of the intersection of health information technology and informed consent, and Heyman (2010) for a rare account of the effects of health IT on solo practices.

9. Aviation, which has been a source of inspiration to those studying the causes and prevention of medical error, also deals with the question of technology-mediated skill degradation. In an airplane, it seems, autopilot tools reduce the ability of pilots to "return to manual" or actually fly the plane (Lowy 2011; cf. Hilkevitch 2012; Prinzel et al. 2002). A US Federal Aviation Administration task force has concluded that:

> Increased availability of advanced generation automation for control of the aircraft flight path has greatly increased the crew's ability to more accurately and precisely control the aircraft's flight path. This, along with a desire to more effectively utilize the limited airspaces available, has led to requirements for operators to equip, train, and use this automation in place of traditional hand flying of the aircraft. Required Navigation Performance approaches, departures, sensitive noise monitoring, and Reduced Vertical Separation Minimum airspace are all examples of either discouraged or prohibited manual flying.
>
> Manual flying, however, remains a required skill for today's aviator. In the case of automation not being available or utilized, the successful outcome of the flight depends on the proficiency of the pilot manually manipulating the flight controls.   (Federal Aviation Administration 2011, 32–3)

   It is of at least passing interest that there is apparently nowhere in the aviation literature a defense of the "pilot-passenger" relationship. Passengers, unlike patients, are likely to be indifferent to the relationship, as long as the plane lands safely.

10. The stethoscope and its history are instructive. The device was invented by René Laënnec in 1816, to better auscultate chest sounds in the obese, to protect the modesty of women, and, with longer stethoscopes, to remain at distance from the smell and fleas of some patients (Weinberg 1993). These instruments were initially thought by some as unlikely and inappropriate: The device made its way from Laënnec's France to England, where, in 1834, an anonymous article in *The London Times* announced:

> That [the stethoscope] will ever come into general use notwithstanding its value is extremely doubtful, because its beneficial application requires much time and gives a good bit of trouble to the patient and to the practitioner, and because its hue and character are foreign and opposed to our habits and associations. There is something even ludicrous in the picture of a grave physician proudly listening through a long tube applied to the patient's thorax.

   This prediction is cited in an article on computers in psychiatry that concludes, "Instead of attacking the *idea* of using patient-computer dialogue in clinical care … let us concentrate our efforts on developing programs that work" (Slack 1989, 321, original emphasis).

11. Advice from the Informatics Committee of the American College of Physicians: "Where previously documented clinical information is still accurate and adds to the value of current documentation, this process of 'review/edit and/or attest, and then copy/forward' (hereafter referred to as copy/forward) of specific prior history or findings may improve the accuracy, completeness, and efficiency of documentation. However, these documentation techniques can also be misused, to the detriment of accuracy, high-quality care, and patient safety" (Kuhn et al. 2015, 302).

12. "Update on the Requirement for Instruction in the Responsible Conduct of Research," available at http://grants1.nih.gov/grants/guide/notice-files/NOT-OD-10-019.html.

13. Available at www.rcr.ethics.gc.ca/eng/policy-politique/framework-cadre/#212. The Tri-Agency, building on earlier Tri-Council policy statements, likewise comprises the Canadian Institutes of Health Research, the Natural Sciences and Engineering Research Council of Canada, and the Social Sciences and Humanities Research Council of Canada.

14. Available at www.universitiesuk.ac.uk/highereducation/Documents/2012/TheConcordatToSupportResearch Integrity.pdf.

15. See note 12.

16. As regards collaboration and team science, note the exciting emergence of "citizen science" or crowdsourcing for empirical research. See, e.g., http://dpcpsi.nih.gov/sites/default/files/Citizen_Science_presentation_to_ Coc_Jan31.pdf; and www.citizensciencealliance.org/.

17. The idea of including biomedical software engineering in the RCR curriculum is due to Dr. Richard Bookman at the University of Miami Miller School of Medicine. Much of this discussion is shaped by discussions with him, for which I am grateful. Dr. Bookman also had the idea of introducing bioscience graduate students to fundamentals of epistemology. I have also enjoyed and benefited from discussions with Greg Wilson, the founder of Software Carpentry. Any errors of fact or failures of analysis remain mine.

18. We are now seeing the emergence of a new kind of forensic statistics, useful for both finding errors in "discoveries" made too quickly and identifying shortcomings in results lacking transparency. The point is not, as in legal forensic statistics, to identify misconduct, but, rather, to correct or illuminate. See, e.g., Wang et al. (2013).

19. See Goldman (1987) and Goodman (1993). When the polio vaccine was announced in 1955, the journalist Edward R. Murrow on the live "See It Now," news program asked the virologist Jonas Salk, "Who owns the patent on this vaccine?" Salk: "Well, the people, I would say. There is no patent. Could you patent the sun?" And he grinned as if he'd heard the punchline of a good joke. (See http://en.wikiquote.org/wiki/Jonas_Salk. Also: "I feel that the greatest reward for success is the opportunity to do more." Cf. Palmer (2014).) A scientist who took a similar position today would be regarded as a chump, a fool, a mystic who did not understand that people will refuse to or cannot do useful and creative work unless financial incentives are dangled in front of them.

20. We must be careful with the use of the terms "replicate," "reproduce," and "corroborate." To replicate an experiment is to do the same experiment, where "same" will range across instruments, reagents, altitude above sea level, and so on. "Reproduce" usually refers to findings. In fact, we might not reproduce others' findings as much as generate evidence in support of them. The term "corroborate" is what therefore should be intended and used. There is much work to be done on distinctions among these three concepts. I am grateful to Dr. Joana Namorado of the European Commission's Directorate for Research and Innovation for insightful discussions of these issues.

21. Thus: http://software-carpentry.org/. Software Carpentry's workshops are attended by students in biomedical research, physics, astronomy, engineering, economics, and other sciences. From an FAQ: "Software Carpentry is a volunteer organization whose goal is to make scientists more productive, and their work more reliable, by teaching them basic computing skills. Founded in 1998, it runs short, intensive workshops that cover program design, version control, testing, and task automation." Software Carpentry has pilot-tested the inclusion of an RCR component in workshops at the University of Miami; that "experiment" is evolving. See also Wilson et al. (2014) for a survey of "best practices for scientific computing." The article was identified as the most-viewed *PLOS Biology* paper of 2014.

22. The "some" in this sentence is crucial and intended to suggest, if not make the point, that it would be a mistake if translational bioscience damaged or impeded basic research, i.e., inquiry motivated or inspired by epistemic curiosity and not a desire to produce a clinical or marketable deliverable.

Chapter 5

Safety, standards, and interoperability

The history of all technologies is in part the story of things that have gone wrong. Some of the history of applied ethics involves how best to prevent and repair those errors. This chapter makes clear the relationship between errors – which can harm people – and ethics, especially in the context of large and complex health information technology systems. From demands for "meaningful use" to disappointment over failures of interoperability, we face many and difficult economic, political, and social challenges. Sometimes the ethics component, it is argued, can be comparably easy.

Errors and their prevention

The dramatic and increasingly rapid expansion of the adoption and use of electronic health records and, to a lesser extent, personal health records has produced a phenomenon replicated time and again in the history of technology: The development and use of an exciting new tool has utterly outstripped the ethical and legal resources required to ensure its appropriate use. From cardiopulmonary resuscitation and organ transplantation to assisted reproductive technology and genetic engineering, the lesson is learned anew with such frequency that one might reasonably wonder why there is such a consistently grand and unsettling disparity between the utensils of science and the customs needed to govern their use.

Moreover, the history of all technologies is in part told in the stories of things that have gone wrong. Error, at least in general, emerges paradoxically as both unavoidable and preventable, and error reduction becomes a moral imperative. The demands of governments and other organizations that health information technology developers and users demonstrate their systems and applications meet criteria for "meaningful use" inherit a tradition of demands for system evaluation as an ethical issue; recall Chapter 2. This presents keen challenges given that most systems were created for scheduling and billing at least as much as for patient care, decision support, and research.

The goal in what follows here is to explore the concept of a "standard" and the circumstances under which standards should be enforced; make clear how error, safety and quality intersect as *ethical* issues; and to conclude with an elaboration of the idea that failure to achieve interoperability is blameworthy, at least, and, at worst, is a betrayal of the very patients we thought we were supposed to be serving.[1]

Standards, error, safety, quality, and interoperability become hinges or levers that allow us to see how human values can and should shape human enterprise, including the design and manufacture of electronic health records. This will set the stage for Chapter 6, which identifies some of the duties of health information technology system makers and vendors and argues for a patient-centered industry.

"Precautions so imperative" – the case of tugboat radios

Where do standards come from?

The tugboats T.J. Hooper and Montrose were towing barges off the New Jersey coast. They both sank during a storm in March 1928 and the cargo that they carried was lost. The owners of the cargo sued the tugboat owners for negligence because they had not equipped the boats with radios that could have provided a warning of the coming storm. Appellate Judge Learned Hand, in a noteworthy legal opinion about the adoption of new technology, agreed:

> An adequate receiving set suitable for a coastwise tug can now be got at small cost and is reasonably reliable if kept up; obviously it is a source of great protection to their tows. Twice every day they can receive these predictions, based upon the widest possible information, available to every vessel within two or three hundred miles and more. Such a set is the ears of the tug to catch the spoken word, just as the master's binoculars are her eyes to see a storm signal ashore ... Indeed in most cases reasonable prudence is in fact common prudence; but strictly it is never its measure; a whole calling may have unduly lagged in the adoption of new and available devices. It never may set its own tests, however persuasive be its usages. Courts must in the end say what is required; there are *precautions so imperative* that even their universal disregard will not excuse their omission.[2]

That is, the tugboat owners were negligent despite that the use of radios had not yet been established as a standard. Put differently, it *should* have been the standard and *should* have been adopted even though the majority of others had not yet done so *and even though there was yet no legal requirement*. If life, limb, and property are on the line, why would one ever want to delay in taking precautions that would protect them?

This might seem counterintuitive to those fledged or who practice under standard-of-care rules that provide some immunity for being in sync with others similarly situated. This is perhaps because this community standard is generally invoked when a physician, say, does not deliver a treatment already known to be effective or misses a diagnosis that a reasonable and prudent colleague would not have missed. To assign responsibility in a case without precedent is overarchingly an *ethical* finding. Judge Hand got it right here, thus helping to make the point that ethics precedes the law (a point emphasized throughout this book).

Undergirding these cases is the notion that an individual can be held responsible for reasonably foreseeable harms. This works well enough in specific cases, but we too often see industries and technologies evolve in such a way that no individual is in a position to prevent a harm, foreseeable or not. The Great Baltimore Fire of 1904 is another important example. The growth of the modern city and the spread of the Industrial Revolution introduced indoor plumbing and citywide pipe networks to deliver water. Fire hydrants were patented devices with varying designs for hose connection threads. Indeed, "Differences in hose connections on the hydrants, both diameters and threads, were part of the design that protected manufacturers from competition" (Seck and Evans 2004, 1). This was doubtless good business, until someone dropped a cigar or cigarette in a sidewalk grate connected to the basement of the John Hurst & Company dry goods store. Some 30 hours later, downtown Baltimore was gone, with more than 1,500 buildings and 2,500 businesses destroyed. Help in the form of fire companies was sent from Washington, D.C., New York, Philadelphia, and other cities. Many were useless, however, as their hoses had different proprietary threads and did not fit Baltimore hydrants.

To be sure, the National Board of Fire Underwriters and the National Fire Protection Association had "advocated a national standard of threads for hoses and fire hydrant outlets before the Great Baltimore Fire, but it received little support" (ibid., 2–3). We do not know how the hose and hydrant lobby responded to these and subsequent efforts at standardization. Doubtless some decried the chilling effect such standards would have on their hose-thread design creativity; perhaps some wept in fury at the idea that big government might stifle hose innovation. In the two decades after the Baltimore fire, the number of cities to adopt standards for size and threading increased steadily, but "Some of the cities made the change only after they experienced their own major fire" (ibid., 3). That is, the risk of this lack of standards and this failure of interoperability were foreseen, but there were no individuals or corporations to hold to account.

Had one of the hose makers designed a faulty hose, there would have been a locus of responsibility. But if hundreds of hose makers made good but incompatible hoses, it becomes the system that is faulty. In this respect, "system" must somehow include or make reference to those who object to or block efforts at standardization.

Why standards?

Civilization's first widely accepted standard was arguably the calendar, which evolved as better means were discovered to predict the change of seasons and to remain useful year after year with greater accuracy.[3] One adopts a calendar out of enlightened self-interest. If it is a good standard, it will make life better, perhaps also easier. But this is a complex affair, and those with an interest in standards might have other interests as well. There is, for instance, money to be made if an individual or a corporation can create or establish a standard that others follow. And others will follow if (i) it serves their purposes, (ii) there is no better alternative, or (iii) they are compelled to.

If "standard" is construed broadly enough, however, calendars must surely lag behind numbering systems themselves or, rather, systems for representing numbers – and these are of a kind with the evolution of alphabets or ideographs. Written languages, be they of alphabet or ideograph, depend on orthographic standards. (Spoken language evolved naturally, like species and their body parts and functions. For a sound to be useful there must be consistency between and among successive utterances, a kind of evolved semantic and syntactic standardization.) The standards we care about here require a decision, an agreement, or a stipulation. Now, there are many reasons for standards. The history of civilization might be cast in part as the discovery and application of standards: plant crops in a row, use this clay for good bricks, divide the year into 12 months ... behave this way and not that, the meter is this long,[4] railroad tracks are this wide ... protect confidentiality with these kinds of encryption algorithms, structure blood gas representations so someone else at another institution can easily obtain and make sense of them, test and validate software this way ... and so on.

We have standards for manufacturing cricket bats and pacemakers, for behaving at funerals, for resecting tumors, for determining who crossed the line first, for how best to catch an anchovy. We use standards for good clinical practice and for protecting human subjects (cf. Institute of Medicine 2001 and its standards for standards for protecting subjects, which amount, in fact, to ethics); and we have standards for people who make standards (and a Society for Standards Professionals, which promotes such standards[5]). Some standards have evolved informally; some were established after debate, and some after a great deal of debate. Some are laws. Some standards address social custom, some help us get through the day without death or disability, and others structure communication media. We should always be about the task of refining or improving all of them, or, at least, those that matter the most. The history of business and industry is in part a history of standardization. Efforts to suppress, avoid, or frustrate standardization usually fail, and with good reason.

Reasons and good reasons

To be a standard is somewhere between a principle or value and a set of criteria, "a set of specifications to which all elements of product, processes, formats, or procedures under its jurisdiction must conform" (Tassey 2000). David and Steinmueller identify four kinds of standards: reference standards, minimum quality standards, technical interface design standards, and compatibility standards. Compatibility standards "assure the user that a component or sub-system can successfully be incorporated, and be 'inter-operable' with other constituents of a large system of closely specified inputs and outputs"(David and Steinmueller, 1994, 218; quoted by Williams et al. 2004, who also cite Tassey; cf. Bredillet 2003).

At a minimum, standards require a reliable way to represent that which is to be standardized. This is an interesting problem in that if we read it incorrectly, it requires there be a standard for the thing to be standardized. Consider St. Isidore of Seville (*c.* 560– *c.* 636), who famously said that melodies "cannot be written."[6] Though he was wrong – there had been earlier and not wholly unsuccessful efforts to transcribe musical notes – what his skepticism illustrates is that getting to the first standard in a domain seems to embed or entail a sense of where it is one wants to arrive. This is a creative undertaking, a kind of bootstrapping. Once the first standard has been articulated, it can be refined and otherwise improved. Indeed, it might even be that a standard-setting project goes off in the wrong direction altogether, requiring more or less extensive correction. The cubit was a great idea, but the ancient Egyptians could not have built pyramids until there was agreement on a standardized cubit rod.

A thorough analysis of the historical, epistemological, and ethical foundations of standards would be a beautiful thing, and a useful project. Pending that, we must focus not on standards *simpliciter* (there are, it seems, standards for certain kinds of push pins), but rather on why we value them in the world of health information technology. First, create a list of reasons for standards and then sort them; then identify which ones are of importance. Here is such a first-approximation list, in no particular order:

- convenience, economy
- reliability, efficiency
- safety
- profit maximization
- values protection, promotion
- quality
- interoperability
- market-share consolidation for early adopters

There are many relationships between and among them – for instance, convenience is unlikely to correlate with values protection; reliability and safety are related, but not always; reliability and efficiency can support cost-control, which we prize; and if we define all the terms properly, quality and interoperability are inseparable. A thorough analysis would identify more, and justify them, and there are likely to be other reasons to add to the list. Some will carry more weight than others; some, but not all, reasons are good reasons. What this means for a project in ethics and informatics is that we can dismiss efficiency, say, as a target of analysis unless it bears in some way on an issue of special interest in informatics ethics.[7] What is wanted here, in informatics, is, in an important if vague respect, what is wanted everywhere in the world of standards: We want to be as good as we can be, along with our efforts and tools, and to improve. That part of "standard" that implies regularity or consistency captures the intuitions that order is more successful than chaos, and that clarity and order produce goods and services that are easier to explain and share. We have something very important to accomplish in health information technology, and good standards are necessary for the process.

Health Level Seven (HL7), arguably the queen of health information technology standards by virtue of its high-quality products and the fact they are freely available, provides many examples of well-wrought standards. One which captures many of the aspects of standards such as are wanted here is the "Electronic Health Record System Functional Model Scope,"[8] an example of what Brooks had in mind when he wrote "conceptual integrity is *the* most important consideration in system design" (1995, 42; original emphasis; cited in and q.v. Russell 2014).

The problem of many standards

That said, anyone who has tried to draft a standard knows how complex the task can be. This is true for fire hoses and railroad tracks, and especially so for the tools of information technology. This is how the International Organization for Standardization (ISO)[9] begins to cast standard "ISO 18308:2011 Health informatics – Requirements for an electronic health record architecture":

> This International Standard defines the set of requirements that shall be met by the architecture of systems and services processing, managing and communicating electronic health record (EHR) information. This is in order to ensure that these EHRs are faithful to the needs of healthcare delivery, are clinically valid and reliable, are ethically sound, meet prevailing legal requirements, support good clinical practice and facilitate data analysis for a multitude of purposes.[10]

This is to promise a great deal. Indeed, to try to ensure (not promote, foster, encourage, support, or salute) "ethical soundness" is a very large project indeed, and a lot to expect even of a well-crafted standard. It is nevertheless a good example of how difficult it is to frame the scope of a standard or define its universe of applicability.

Moreover, the standards cosmology is vast, so much so that for some purposes there is more than one "standard" – itself an interesting concept. (A popular witticism in the health information technology community suggests that "The great thing about medical informatics standards is that there are so many to choose from." That it is well known is itself a source of interest.) Of the reasons for standards itemized just above, any one of them might be linked to ethics: Efficiency reduces waste, always a virtue; quality can entail keeping a promise; and so on. Here, we care most about three: values protection and promotion, safety, and interoperability.

Regarding the first, what is meant is that values such as privacy and confidentiality can be, and are, supported by a variety of standards; the same is true for security, which comprises part of any system for protecting privacy and confidentiality. As earlier, the literally most compelling privacy standard is the law; in the United States, for instance, there are 51 such standards, one for each state, and the federal Privacy Rule under HIPAA; indeed, one of the virtues of HIPAA was an attempt to set a national "floor" of privacy protections to harmonize the legal Babel resulting from 50 different laws in an age in which health information was flowing across state boundaries. Health care institutions are subject to both the federal law and the applicable state law, whichever is more rigorous. There are several privacy standards. The ISO has developed some (including ISO/TS 14441:2013, "Health informatics – Security and privacy requirements of EHR systems for use in conformity assessment"; and ISO/DTR 18638, "Components of Education to Ensure Health Information Privacy"); (ISO/TS 25237:2008, "Health informatics – Pseudonymization"); and others address privacy and security in non-health domains. Health Level Seven International[11] has developed several (including "HL7 Version 3 Standard: Security and Privacy Ontology, Release 1," "HL7 Healthcare Privacy and Security Classification System," and "HL7 Version 3 Standard: Privacy, Access and Security Services." Compare the ASTM's[12] E1869-04(2014)) "Standard Guide for Confidentiality, Privacy, Access, and Data Security Principles for Health Information Including Electronic Health Records; and ASTM E2473-05(2011) "Standard Practice for the Occupational/Environmental Health View of the Electronic Health Record." Others address information security, data transmission, laboratory systems, dentistry, and so on.

The question how a responsible institution should sort this out is complex, difficult and, apparently, the preserve of consulting firms. Much the same has occurred in the law in some jurisdictions. The relationship between HIPAA and each state law, for instance, has been fodder for a number of white papers and proprietary analyses. (At its inception, HIPAA was thought by some to be a kind of full-employment act for consultants. The observation was neither snide nor snarky: Unlike all other ethics policies, which are generally, under Joint Commission guidelines, to be the work of institutional ethics committees, US hospital privacy policies were overwhelmingly the work of outside consultants and law firms.) Sorting this out will not be our task here; moreover, we have perhaps spent adequate time on privacy and confidentiality in Chapter 3.

We earlier emphasized three primary reasons for standards: values protection, safety, and interoperability. The first led to a survey of privacy standards. But safety and interoperability go to the very core of why we want to evolve from paper health records to electronic health records in the first place.

We are searching here for longer reach and a surer grasp of the role of standards in supporting those values that matter the most. Let us assume that the world wants better electronic health records and data interchange; and the reason for that is the well-founded belief that such improvements will improve health care, which will, in turn, lengthen lives and reduce human suffering – and do so reliably and affordably. What we want is to avoid relearning the lessons of tugboat radios, that is, we seek to have the structure and function of a crucial industry or service section clear enough so that every player or agent sees what precautions are imperative and, consequently, takes them. A pair of findings from an influential report by JASON, an independent scientific advisory group, points in this direction:

- "Although current efforts to define standards for EHRs and to certify HIT systems are useful, they lack a unifying software architecture to support broad interoperability. Interoperability is best achieved through the development of a comprehensive, open architecture."

- "Current approaches for structuring EHRs and achieving interoperability have largely failed to open up new opportunities for entrepreneurship and innovation that can lead to products and services that enhance health care provider workflow and strengthen the connection between the patient and the health care system, thus impeding progress toward improved health outcomes" (JASON 2014, 40)[13]

The report recommends the US Office of the National Coordinator for Health Information Technology (ONC), created in 2004 and which has struggled to improve data interchange and interoperability,[14] "define an overarching software architecture for the health data infrastructure" (ibid.).[15]

There is an eerie parallel between the competing ideas of standards and open architectures. The former must be agreed to, perhaps under incentives, or stipulated, perhaps by law. If electronic health record vendors and users refuse to adopt the standards then, absent a legal impetus, there is nothing to be done; this is much the situation we have today. JASON recommends that open architectures be based on "application program interfaces" that should be "certified through vetting by multiple third-party developers in regularly scheduled 'code-athons'" (ibid., 7), and that the architectures be agnostic as to type, scale, platform, and storage location of the data (ibid., 26). Significantly:

> The architecture must be based on open standards and published application program interfaces (APIs) and protocols. Standards, APIs, and protocols all aim to achieve the same basic outcome, which is to enable the seamless interaction among components. To achieve interoperability for EHRs and to open the entrepreneurial space for software development, all of these elements must be made public. People frequently encounter standards in their daily lives. For example, an E26 light bulb has a standard base diameter and conductor position to allow mating with a compatible socket, which also has standard properties. One uses different names for this same basic concept at different levels. The term "standard" typically is used for basic components, especially those that have a physical instantiation or interaction. Standards usually are established through a formal process and are endorsed by a standards organization, such as the IEEE, ISO, or ANSI. There are hundreds of such organizations, most of which are centered on a particular industry. In contrast, an API is seldom a standard and is usually dictated by a vendor.   (ibid., 26–7)

If the makers of electronic health records need not hew to standards, and if we have yet to develop adequate open-source application program interfaces, then it is not clear how or when we will attain the level of interoperability reckoned necessary to ensure safety and high quality.

The US Health Information Technology for Economic and Digital Health (HITECH) Act was passed in 2009 to stimulate the use of electronic records. It included financial incentives – $19 billion in financial incentives – to foster "meaningful use" in various stages. It applied to individual institutions, which went into dervish-like motions to attest to the fact that they were, indeed, using their new electronic records meaningfully. Indeed, individual institutions saw improvement (Encinosa and Bae 2015). Unhappily, although this stimulated the economy, and generated splendid business for makers and vendors of electronic health records, it did not improve our ability to exchange health information.[16]

If safety and interoperability are to be secured, systems will need to identify a comprehensive set of standards, protocols, rules, policies, and best practices covering the following:[17]

- use of electronic health records data for clinical care, research, public health and epidemiologic research, decision support, and quality assessment

- interinstitutional data exchange and participation in health information exchanges
- patient access to electronic health records
- interactions between and among electronic health records and personal health records
- role of electronic health records in managing the communication of incidental findings (as result from any of the above)
- software validation and performance and conformance testing

This task is gargantuan. Worse, it must address and overcome electronic health record vendors' objections to external requirements to foster interoperability, an issue to be taken up in the next chapter. What is wanted is nothing less than an evolution in the "standard of care" for the adoption of standards. The challenge before us here is not to assess when the standard of care for electronic health records use or governance has shifted or become established, or to identify and endorse the best way to do these things. It is, rather, to take stock at this crucial juncture of the ethical underpinnings of standards themselves.

Here is a modest proposal: Those organizations offering prizes for innovative products, Turing machines, and the like might consider the following social experiment. They should fund a comparison of the three best-known open-source electronic health records with those of the three largest vendors. Compare the systems based on audits of user satisfaction (including ease of use, functionality, and screen design), decision support system accuracy, and security. This would, of course, require the vendors to grant licenses for copies of their software packages and other components. With appropriate and adequate confidentiality agreements, surely the vendors would agree to participate.

Electronic health records as a "disruptive technology"

Electronic health record systems are, and mass-produced automobiles were, "disruptive technologies" or "disruptive innovations." The latter supplanted horse-drawn buggies and the former are in the process of replacing paper medical records. Electronic health records also have created a market; there is very little money to be made in the paper, folders, and binders used to hold records, whereas automobiles killed the buggy industry.

The business theorist Clayton M. Christensen, who first used the phrase "disruptive technologies" (Bower and Christensen 1995), is a source of advice for businesses seeking to retain market share. As much as anything, the concept of disruptive technologies is used by businesses to preserve preeminence, in part because successful, well-run firms that prize customer service are especially vulnerable to the next disruptive competitor (Christensen 1997). Disruptive competition leads to lower performance by existing businesses because it protects customers who are not very demanding.

We lack a good history of the EHR industry. Most of the advances in electronic health record use and development have been academic and/or fostered with government support. Whereas entities that need and use electronic health records will insist they are "patient-centric," the firms that make them and sell consulting services to operate them have never needed to attend to patients as much as to the hospitals buying their systems. Those hospitals, we hypothesize, are for the most part prepared to endure "good enough" electronic health record systems. In addition to this is the impossibility of direct comparisons and hence valid competition between and among vendors, leading to a race to a lowest-common-denominator level of service. Electronic health records end up as just good enough, too. When "good enough" is widespread, market share is preserved.[18] This might explain why, for all the economic motivation provided to the electronic health record industry, there is so little bona fide competition, and product quality is often so very disappointing.

Interoperability as an ethical issue

The health care division of a very well-known international technology company manufactures a fetal monitor, or device for measuring fetal heart rates. The firm also manufactures electronic health record systems. Hospital Alpha uses this monitor, but it has in place a competing electronic health record. The monitor's output or heart tracings can be viewed on a screen and printed, but the only way to capture these data for the competing EHR is to print the tracings, scan them, and upload them.

If this were any other industry, such a state of affairs would be both laughable and intolerable. Imagine someone in the financial service industry having to print, scan, and upload reports if received on a different e-mail system, or different tracks for different trains, different hoses for different hydrants, or different radios to listen to different stations. In health care, however, there is little that is laughable in failure to make patient care safe, effective, and efficient. In the same way it has been documented that health budget increases can be linked to lower mortality rates (Sommers et al. 2012), there is an opportunity to conduct an analysis to demonstrate that improved interoperability likewise leads to reduced mortality or, if one prefers, there being fewer dead people.

The interoperability of electronic health records should not be a market strategy, a bonus for loyal customers, or an inducement to obtain new customers. It is a moral obligation that accompanies the care of patients and biomedical research in the twenty-first century. Failure to achieve interoperability becomes a moral failure.

This is not a duty for individual physicians and nurses, although they could have been more compelling in demanding that the tools they use work better; and it is not immediately an obligation for individual hospitals or other health care institutions, despite that they have, ensemble, mysteriously been willing to pay vast sums for mediocre systems that do not communicate with each other. As with any other product, any shortcomings in design or manufacturer lie with the designers or manufacturers. In the absence of their willingness to improve lifesaving and life-prolonging products, it is the duty of society to require that they do.

This is emphatically not intended to constitute an argument for increased government regulation (although if that is the only means to achieve life-saving improvements, so be it). It is rather an attempt to recognize the internal excellence and evolving commitment of designers and manufacturers and to suggest to them, as we have always done for all industries, that enlightened self-interest can point the way to interoperability. It is enlightened in that it will enable them to do the right thing for the right reason, and self-interested in that firms that embrace interoperability will be recognized and praised for their effort. There are many ways for electronic health record vendors to compete that do not require giving away the family secrets.

Here is a simple example: Standard electronic health record implementations do not include useful or helpful tools for documenting end-of-life preferences. At most is a 0/1 switch indicating whether a patient should receive full resuscitation attempts in the event of cardiopulmonary failure. That's it: code or no-code. Nothing about supporting documentation such as links to living wills, DNR orders, and the communication that should usually precede a DNR,[19] or designations of a health care surrogate to direct treatment in the event of a patient's incapacity. Given that hospital ethics committees spend a great deal of time on end-of-life care and associated policies, this is a potentially fertile opportunity for such committees to be included more in the activities of information technology units. Hospitals around the country are retrofitting their off-the-shelf electronic health record systems to attend to this crucial and delicate component of the care of dying or very sick patients (cf. Bhatia et al. 2015; Sulmasy and Marx 1997). It would be easy for electronic health record vendors to design nimble end-of-life functions or apps, and, moreover, make them electronically portable or, if you will, interoperable, with each other and with online advance-directive repositories. Then it will be a little more possible for these firms to compete on the basis of usability and price – as other industries do all the time. Copyright screen shots if necessary, guard clever code if one must – but please do not make it difficult to determine what is to be done if a patient's heart stops.

The inadequacies and failures of paper records included risks to patient safety, and so electronic records became a means to protect patients (see, e.g., Jha and Classen 2011). The ethical warrant for improving safety and interoperability is overwhelmingly utilitarian. Indeed, the utilitarian basis for this claim has been tacit throughout. It will benefit many, have little or no collateral damage, and meets no good counterexample. It is also, we might say, a way to demonstrate our commitments to patients, to treat them with respect, to place their interests above all others, even if this means reduced quarterly earnings. It is therefore also what must be done under any of several rule-and-rights-based or deontological moral systems. For that matter, and unlike many other challenges in health care and bioethics, the duty to achieve (improved) interoperability is ethically simple and straightforward.

Notes

1. I am grateful to Kimberly Loveland for her work on a document annotating some of the material in this chapter.

2. *In re* Eastern Transportation Co. (The T.J. Hooper), 60 F.2d 737 (2d Cir. 1932), pp. 739–40, emphasis added. The case is sometimes cited by scholars in the health information technology community (cf. Berner 2002; Epstein 1992). Judge Hand is also the source of a subsequent and important balancing test used to determine negligence: *United States* v. *Carroll Towing Co.* 159 F.2d 169 (2d Cir. 1947).

3. See the American National Standards Institute (ANSI) précis on standards through history, www.ansi.org/consumer_affairs/history_standards.aspx?menuid=5.

4. The history of the meter as a standard is a favorite example of the difficulties in getting all this just right. According to the (US) National Institute of Science and Technology (where the United States, along with Liberia and Myanmar, has yet to adopt the metric system):

   The origins of the meter go back to at least the 18th century. At that time, there were two competing approaches to the definition of a standard unit of length. Some suggested defining the meter as the length of a pendulum having a half-period of one second; others suggested defining the meter as one ten-millionth of the length of the earth's meridian along a quadrant (one fourth the circumference of the earth). In 1791, soon after the French Revolution, the French Academy of Sciences chose the meridian definition over the [English] pendulum definition because the force of gravity varies slightly over the surface of the earth, affecting the period of the pendulum.

Thus, the meter was intended to equal 10^{-7} or one ten-millionth of the length of the meridian through Paris from pole to the equator. However, the first prototype was short by 0.2 millimeters because researchers miscalculated the flattening of the earth due to its rotation. Still this length became the standard. In 1889, a new international prototype was made of an alloy of platinum with 10 percent iridium, to within 0.0001, that was to be measured at the melting point of ice. In 1927, the meter was more precisely defined as the distance, at 0°, between the axes of the two central lines marked on the bar of platinum-iridium kept at the [Bureau International des Poids et Mesures], and declared Prototype of the meter by the 1st [Conférence Générale des Poids et Mesures (CGPM)], this bar being subject to standard atmospheric pressure and supported on two cylinders of at least one centimeter diameter, symmetrically placed in the same horizontal plane at a distance of 571 mm from each other.

The 1889 definition of the meter, based upon the artifact international prototype of platinum-iridium, was replaced by the CGPM in 1960 using a definition based upon a wavelength of krypton-86 radiation. This definition was adopted in order to reduce the uncertainty with which the meter may be realized. In turn, to further reduce the uncertainty, in 1983 the CGPM replaced this latter definition by the following definition:

The meter is the length of the path travelled by light in vacuum during a time interval of 1/299 792 458 of a second. (http://physics.nist.gov/cuu/Units/meter.html; and see www.bipm.org/en/measure ment-units/history-si/evolution-metre.html)

5. www.ses-standards.org/.

6. Actually (remember that "music" comes from "Muses"), what he said was, "The sound of the Muses, since it is a perceptible thing, flows by in a passing moment of time, and is impressed upon the memory. Whence the poets wrote that the Muses were daughters of Jupiter and Memory. Unless sounds are held in a person's memory they perish, because they cannot be written down" (Isidore of Seville 2013, III.15.1).

    An encyclopedist too often overlooked as a precursor to Diderot, d'Alembert, and the French encyclo-pedists of the eighteenth century, Isidore wrote the "Etymologies," which comprise 20 books on topics ranging from grammar, animals, and agriculture to arithmetic, geometry, music, and astronomy.

7. Efficiency will always manage to avoid being nontrivial by its association with resource conservation, waste avoidance, including waste of human effort, and so on. The lack of efficiency can in fact gum up everything. This is just to underscore the importance of definitions in any typology of standards.

8. HL7 EHR-System Functional Model, R2:

    The HL7 EHR-S Functional Model defines a standardized model of the functions that may be present in EHR Systems. From the outset, a clear distinction between the EHR as a singular entity and systems that operate on the EHR – i.e., EHR Systems is critical. ... Notably, the EHR-S Functional Model does not address whether the EHR-S is a system-of-systems or a single system providing the functions required by the users. This standard makes no distinction regarding implementation – the EHR-S described in a Functional Profile may be a single system or a system of systems. Within the normative sections of the Functional Model, the term "system" is used generically to cover the continuum of implementation options. This includes "core" healthcare functionality, typically provided by health-care-specific applications that manage electronic healthcare information. It also includes associated generic application-level capabilities that are typically provided by middleware or other infrastruc-ture components. The latter includes interoperability and integration capabilities such as location discovery and such areas as cross application workflow. Interoperability is considered both from semantic (clear, consistent and persistent communication of meaning) and technical (format, syntax and physical connectivity) viewpoints. Further, the functions make no statement about which technology is used, or about the content of the electronic health record.

    Finally, the EHR-S Functional Model supports research needs by ensuring that the data available to researchers follow the required protocols for privacy, confidentiality, and security. The diversity of research needs precludes the specific listing of functions that are potentially useful for research. (www.hl7.org/implement/standards/product_brief.cfm?product_id=269)

9. The ISO, which has published more than 19,500 international standards, has this acronym "Because 'International Organization for Standardization' would have different acronyms in different languages

(IOS in English, OIN in French for *Organisation internationale de normalisation*), our founders decided to give it the short form ISO. ISO is derived from the Greek isos, meaning equal ..." (www.iso.org/iso/home/about.htm).

10. It continues:

This International Standard defines the set of requirements that shall be met by the architecture of systems and services processing, managing and communicating electronic health record (EHR) information. This is in order to ensure that these EHRs are faithful to the needs of healthcare delivery, are clinically valid and reliable, are ethically sound, meet prevailing legal requirements, support good clinical practice and facilitate data analysis for a multitude of purposes.

For the purposes of this International Standard, the EHR is defined as:

"one or more repositories, physically or virtually integrated, of information in computer proces-sable form, relevant to the wellness, health and healthcare of an individual, capable of being stored and communicated securely and of being accessible by multiple authorized users, represented according to a standardized or commonly agreed logical information model. Its primary purpose is the support of life-long, effective, high quality and safe integrated healthcare."

To complement this definition, the ideal vision of health (and consequently health information) is reflected in the WHO definition from 1946:

"Health is a state of complete physical, mental and social well-being and not merely the absence of disease or infirmity."

The scope of the EHR is recognized as being broader than the documentation of illnesses and their prevention and treatment. The systems and services that are deemed potential contributors to an EHR will increasingly include systems capturing complementary therapy, wellness, and home care information in addition to the conventional clinical systems within healthcare provider organizations. (www.iso.org/obp/ui/#iso:std:iso:18308:ed-1:v1:en; note omitted).

11. "Level Seven" refers to the "seventh level of the International Organization for Standardization (ISO) seven-layer communications model for Open Systems Interconnection (OSI) – the application level. The application level interfaces directly to and performs common application services for the application processes. Although other protocols have largely superseded it, the OSI model remains valuable as a place to begin the study of network architecture" (www.hl7.org/about/index.cfm?ref=nav).

12. Formerly the American Society for Testing and Materials.

13. This report includes a positive and refreshing take on the role of clinicians and others in health information technology: "Despite cynicism about the US health care system, the 878,000 licensed physicians, 2.8 million registered nurses, and nearly 10 million other medical professionals are focused primarily on caring for their patients. When faced with decisions about how to implement systems for exchanging health information, one should ask: 'What is best for the patient?' The answer usually provides clarity to help cut through the debate about these matters" (JASON 2014, 29). The report also emphasizes the importance of the role of patient trust in health information systems.

JASON, which has traditionally received funding through the US Department of Defense, does not publish the names of the scientists who contribute to its reports.

14. www.healthit.gov/newsroom/about-onc. The organization maintains a robust privacy office but has so far disdained any substantive interest in ethics in informatics construed more broadly.

15. ONC interoperability initiatives comprise CONNECT (www.healthit.gov/policy-researchers-implementers/connect-gateway-nationwide-health-information-network) and DIRECT (www.healthit.gov/policy-researchers-implementers/direct-project).

16. Stage 1 and 2 Meaningful Use standards "fall short of achieving meaningful use in any practical sense. At present, large-scale interoperability amounts to little more than replacing fax machines with the electronic delivery of page-formatted medical records. Most patients still cannot gain electronic access to their health information. Rational access to EHRs for clinical care and biomedical research does not exist outside the boundaries of individual organizations" (JASON 2014, 6).

17. Standards for interoperability are thought through most clearly and usefully in HL7's "Fast Healthcare Interoperability Resources," or FHIR; see http://hl7.org/implement/standards/fhir/summary.html.

18. A related concept is too pretty to be left. Karl Marx speculated that periodic economic crises were an essential component of capitalism, which needed constantly to identify new sources of wealth production. "Creative destruction" – a term later coined by others – was needed to manufacture crises to clear the way for the bourgeois to realize new means of wealth acquisition. See Elliott (1978).

19. For instance, as required for Physician Orders for Life-Sustaining Treatment, or POLST for www.polst.org.

The e-health industry
Markets, vendors, and regulators

Electronic health records are big business, and the companies that make and sell them are big businesses. Unlike traditional pharmaceutical and medical device manufacturers, the developers and makers of electronic health records are so far and for the most part immune to scrutiny and regulation. Accounts of vendors discouraging unmediated error reports and other forms of clinician-to-clinician communication and restricting the kinds of comparative analysis that has driven scientific progress in other health industries point to a need to assess the appropriate roles and responsibilities of vendors. Duties of system manufacturers and vendors are considered along with corporate responsibility in a free market, and the role of ethics in sorting out duties. Included in this assessment is a discussion of the ethically and conceptually interesting questions whether electronic health records and their accoutrements are medical devices and whether they should be regulated.

Health care and the marketplace

The idea, the very idea, that the services of clinicians and hospitals might have market value is of comparatively recent vintage. For most of history, the practice of medicine, for instance, was something undertaken by professionals at distance from market forces. Taking care of the sick was just what one did, in exchange for whatever one was given, which was often little or nothing. By the same token, for most of history, little or nothing in the medical armamentarium worked, or worked very well. A talented physician or surgeon with a good reputation could command fees, if not higher fees, for middling results. By the turn of the nineteenth century, the idea that physicians might be motivated by anything other than prolonging life and ending suffering had become the stuff of stinging calumny. George Bernard Shaw, in the "Preface on Doctors" to his *The Doctor's Dilemma*, is furious:

> It is not the fault of our doctors that the medical service of the community, as at present provided for, is a murderous absurdity. That any sane nation, having observed that you could provide for the supply of bread by giving bakers a pecuniary interest in baking for you, should go on to give a surgeon a pecuniary interest in cutting off your leg, is enough to make one despair of political humanity. But that is precisely what we have done. And the more appalling the mutilation, the more the mutilator is paid. He who corrects the ingrowing toe-nail receives a few shillings: he who cuts your inside out receives hundreds of guineas, except when he does it to a poor person for practice. ... Scandalized voices murmur that these operations are necessary. They may be. It may also be necessary to hang a man or pull down a house. But we take good care not to make the hangman and the housebreaker the judges of that. If we did, no man's neck would be safe and no man's house stable. (Shaw 1909, v)

This mean rant should be part of every conflict-of-interest curriculum.

But Shaw was not merely doctor-bashing. His misanthropy was plenary: "Doctors are just like other Englishmen," the Irishman wrote, "... most of them have no honor and no conscience: what they commonly mistake for these is sentimentality and an intense dread of doing anything that everybody else does not do, or omitting to do anything that everybody else does" (p. viii). Still he, like others, wanted to hold clinicians to a higher standard. There are many good reasons for this, and it is why we try to teach our medical and nursing students that they are not like bakers or hangmen or peddlers. By virtue of their special training, their ancient codes, their social authority, and their patients' lack of it, they must hew to standards shaped by humanistic and not commercial motivations. This is a very high standard, and it is no small task to convince some doctors that they must be self-effacing and altruistic while those who surround them and provide their instruments, drugs, and, now, computers are turning a smart profit.

But what should we say are the moral obligations of those who develop and sell medical devices and pharmaceutical products? While the expectations laid on professionals were never intended to apply to car dealers or greengrocers, there are good reasons to hope that the inventors and/or makers and/or sellers of vaccines, HIV drugs, and pacemakers, say, might be willing to accept duties related to the health of populations, the needs of patients, or even the duties of those who use and prescribe their products. This is related to the issue of supply chain management in business ethics. Consider the food industry (Maloni and Brown 2006). It is not enough to expect and require that a supermarket not make us (immediately) sick with its products – we might also expect and require that the deliverers, farmers, seed producers, and others contribute to the availability of nontoxic or even healthy products. We might even assign them, all of them, responsibility to foster environmental sustainability, not to exploit workers, and so on. We might further want corporations to be socially responsible and therefore to make some products available cheaply or for free to poor people, to support education programs, and to share profits with communities – for instance.

Now consider three of several possible responses to the question whether medical product makers might have duties related to those of clinicians because their products are essential to clinical practice.

First, the health and medical industries owe nothing more to society or humanity than any other businesses do, and that is not very much, if anything. Their duties are to shareholders and investors, who have provided the resources to which the businesses add imagination and industriousness to create valuable products. The moral status of a device that saves a life is indistinguishable from a handkerchief, potato, or carburetor. Let us call this the "libertarian response." Second, medical products, because they are necessary to human health and survival, owe the world the same thing as a physician or nurse – at least some selflessness. People should develop such products for the good they do, not the profits they reap. This is the "altruistic response." A third response makes clear that these sketches of libertarians and altruists are cartoons – that no one but the most ideologically naïve capitalist would seriously defend utterly unfettered markets, and no one with any knowledge of human motivation would think that love of the common good is, alone, adequate inspiration to elicit the sweat of progress. Each system had its shot on goal in the twentieth century and each, in failing, caused immeasurable human misery. (Cf. Francis Fukuyama's discovery of the intellectual failure of neoconservatism and his likening of it to Leninism [Fukuyama 2006].) So this "none-of-the-above" response must somehow hybridize obligations to be self-effacing and place patient interests ahead of others, on the one hand, and, on the other, to recognize the fact that many people are motivated and even inspired by economic self-interest. This is an ancient conflict: individual versus collective, self-interest versus solidarity, rights versus responsibilities.

Our Information Age thrives at a time when the technologies used in hospitals are, generally, developed not by free-acting and creative individualists and not (except, for instance, the US Veterans Administration) by democratic governments. They are developed, manufactured, and sold by international entities that have fiduciary duties to shareholders and investors. Indeed, those corporate duties can themselves be cast as moral obligations. We live in an "investment culture" in which investors or speculators risk stakes on the success of organizations (businesses) which likewise invest vast sums to develop, market, and sell products. These are said to be virtues of free markets.

Conceptually founded in part on the work of Ludwig von Mises and Friedrich Hayek, ex-pats and exports of the Vienna School's bitter anti-Socialism, this celebration of investment economies is undergirded by the straightforward intuition that if one has taken a risk, she is somehow more deserving of a reward. If I have skin in the game, I *deserve* to share in the profit. A consequence of this is what we can call "the racetrack effect" – I study the ponies, pore over their records, calculate or note the odds, and then place a bet. Depending on skill and luck, my investment is either rewarded or it is not. Sometimes skill loses and sometimes luck wins. Now, this is fine for racetracks, but perhaps not so good for economies, in which one's losses often involve other people's money and entail the suffering of those who steer clear of racetracks, casinos, and stock markets, but, unfortunately, were not aware they could lose without placing a bet.

It is worth noting that Hayek, the hero of many contemporary libertarians, held some views utterly at odds with contemporary free marketeers, US "Tea Party" zealots, and privatizers who believe the only legitimate role of government is national defense, law enforcement, and tax breaks for using foreign banks. Hayek defended government-funded "safety nets." He wrote:

> *There is no reason why*, in a society which has reached the general level of wealth ours has, the first kind of security should not be guaranteed to all without endangering general freedom. ... *there can be no doubt* that some minimum of food, shelter and clothing, sufficient to preserve health and the capacity to work, can be assured to everybody. Indeed, for a considerable part of the population of England this sort of security has long been achieved. ... *Nor is there any reason why* the state should not help to organize a comprehensive system of social insurance in providing for those common hazards of life against which few can make adequate provision.
>
> (Hayek 2007, 148; emphasis added)

If one could publish *The Time-Machine Times*, a headline might read, "Libertarian Endorses Obamacare and NHS; Calls for Health-Care Safety Net; Affirms No Threat to Liberty."

In any event, what this means is that our "none-of-the-above" stance, namely, neither libertarian nor altruist, is vulnerable to intense forms of politico-economic buffeting. We are not likely to resolve this issue here (though we do attempt to make the case for patient-centered industry at the end of the chapter). What we can do is seek the kind of touchstones that applied ethics offers and often has provided to responsible businesses. It is guided by the following considerations and assumptions, intended to be uncontroversial:

1. No developer of seller of electronic health records would ever publicly confess, "Our business plan is to acquire vast personal and corporate wealth based on the misfortunes of sick people."
2. Making a profit is a legitimate goal of this and other industries.
3. Fair competition can improve quality and nurture innovation.
4. Even if a business does not adopt all of the components of corporate social responsibility, it is not onerous, unreasonable, or anathema to corporate mission to identify and meet obligations to patients and, more generally, to support the communities that were the sources of profit in the first place.
5. While there are significant differences between patients and investors and between health professionals and corporations – even in the world of electronic patient records[1] – it is also the case that the health care industry is different in kind from others, precisely because patients are not analogous to investors, shareholders, customers, or any such thing.

The touchstones or core principles are likewise uncontroversial, or should be: *transparency, veracity,* and *accountability/responsibility.* In many organizations, these are understood to be components of an overarching stance toward *integrity* and *trust* (discussed in Chapter 4). Now, it should go without saying that these values are not merely to be espoused or endorsed. To trumpet your organization's commitment to these values without incorporating, adopting, or metabolizing them as part of bona fide institutional culture is rather to accept the embrace of hypocrisy (in which case one is not transparent, undermines veracity, and shuns responsibility). In North America, at least, the academic and corporate workplace is increasingly shaped by workshops, intranet "training," and signings of personal statements of commitment to corporate integrity. Some, perhaps much, of this is fostered by the requirements of corporate compliance, which, in turn, is at least sometimes the unhappy offspring of noteworthy criminal cases and instances of dreadful publicity. Make no mistake: An institution might avoid legal charges and front-page embarrassment and still not embrace, sincerely, the tenets of an integrity program. For all the importance of veracity, for instance, the law rarely punishes deception. It could not be otherwise: Imagine a CEO being arrested every time one withheld, stretched, or narrowed the truth. A code of ethics that crows about the company's commitment to "the highest ethical standards" – as if there were layers or levels or grades of ethical standards and we, of course, bought the best one – will do more harm than good if those to whom it is supposed to apply know the boss is hiding something, noodling with the truth, and then shrugging when found out. A "culture of compliance" can be a risky thing if it lacks authenticity; the Enron Corporation had a fine code of ethics, as we saw in Chapter 4, and all employees were required to sign a statement saying they had received a copy.

Transparency

To suggest that a firm that makes and sells electronic health records should hew to standards of corporate transparency is to make a broad and vague claim. Does it require that the firm not have corporate secrets? To answer that question requires further elaboration of what it means to have a legitimate corporate secret. Surely the demands of transparency do not entail disclosure of legitimate trade secrets, but equally surely they do not require that known bugs affecting patient safety be withheld from other users. A useful corporate exercise, perhaps during an ethics workshop, would include a discussion of what sorts of things ought to be disclosed and what sorts may be withheld – and why. Government regulations affecting or requiring business disclosures might be a place to start.

In the United States, for example, beginning with the Truth in Securities Act of 1933, a post-Depression effort to require financial disclosure to investors, and extending to the Sarbanes-Oxley Act of 2002, a recognition of the fact that corporate corruption could destroy an economy, it has been clear that integrity workshops alone are inadequate means of limiting deceit, theft, and fraud. But those workshops might serve to raise awareness of the kinds of decisions that raise ethical issues and about which the law is silent. To teach only what the law forbids and not what morality requires is a facile shorthand that cannot impart the skills of critical thinking required for applied ethics. One way to improve those skills is to hone them on guided discussion of case studies.

There is an important distinction to be drawn between *transparency* and *secrecy*. The former labels an approach or stance to business (or personal) practice. To be transparent is to make it easy to obtain information a reasonable person would want to have before making a decision. The best example of this is in the ethics of informed or valid consent for clinical practice and for research. Recall that the components of valid consent are, generally, (i) adequate information, (ii) voluntariness, and (iii) mental capacity to understand and appreciate the information. Although we might debate what constitutes "adequate information" in a particular case, there should be no disagreement that at a minimum it should include information about risks, benefits, and alternatives of the therapy proposed or the experiment contemplated. In this context, it would be a grievous breach of transparency to fail to disclose the most likely risks.[2] Contemporary attention to conflicts of interest has led to requirements that prospective participants in research studies be told if investigators are receiving payment or other incentives to conduct the trials.

For our purposes, "secrecy" means withholding, concealing, or failing to disclose something from someone or more people. It can be episodic, brief, or long-standing, but, unlike transparency, it is not a general policy or stance. "A path, a riddle, a jewel, an oath – anything can be secret," writes the philosopher Sissela Bok, "so long as it is kept intentionally hidden, set apart in the mind of its keeper as requiring concealment" (Bok 1983, 5). She correctly seeks a neutral definition of "secret" to prevent "evil secrets" from "casting a pall on *all* that is kept secret, including much that stands in no need of being done to death" (p. 9, original emphasis). Keeping some secrets is morally permissible, but that is not the case for some others. It is one thing to conceal a trade secret, and another to conceal the fact that your computer program is designed, say, to make it easy to commit billing fraud.

Even some legitimate secrets do not enjoy plenary justification but must be disclosed to regulators or overseers. Drug formulas might be kept secret from competitors but not the government or bodies overseeing research. Furthermore, having generally or collectively valuable information but neglecting it or preventing access to it is an affront to transparency.

Veracity

Transparency and veracity are intertwined in complex ways. One might disdain transparency for the truths it would reveal or forgo veracity and therefore forfeit transparency. Generally, "veracity" is about communicating the truth as best one can, à la Coleridge: "Veracity does not consist in saying, but in the intention of communicating the truth." This captures the insight that a false utterance is deceptive only if the speaker knows of its falsehood – he might merely be mistaken.

Playing with the truth is an ancient pastime. One might simply lie, or utter something known to be false; remain silent, when speaking would clarify or correct; or even speak a narrow truth with the intention of deceiving: There are four anchovies on a plate in a crowded room, but you, in error, believe there are five. After you leave the room, I eat all the anchovies. Upon your return you ask me, "Did you eat the five anchovies?" I look you in the eye and say, "No! I did not eat the five anchovies." It is true that I did not eat five anchovies; that is, I have uttered a sentence that narrowly corresponds to the facts.[3] I did not eat five anchovies. I ate four, but my intent was to have you believe I ate none. So a good way to think about deception is this: knowingly or recklessly causing or permitting someone to have a false belief. Veracity, as the poet said, just above, is the intention to communicate truthfully. (This discussion underscores the important role of intention in applied ethics, perhaps especially bioethics; see Shaw 2006.)

Even if deception could be justified in special circumstances, as for instance when under duress or to avoid hurting feelings, it is not likely that the manufacturers of medical devices and electronic health records should ever have an occasion in which to depart from the demands of veracity. It is uncontroversially unacceptable to say a system can do things it cannot. It is blameworthy to alter records or data or spreadsheets to prevent bad public relations or erosion in market share. It is wrong to (try to) prevent others from communicating with veracity. Some of these proscriptions are captured in the laws governing markets, security transactions, and public stock offerings. Even some lovers of unfettered markets underscore the importance of reliable information in a free economy. That we have laws governing this is because some businesses were deceptive (among other things), and this damaged the marketplace. Like murder, rape, and armed robbery, this is not ethically very interesting. That is, while any credible system of morality will make clear why murder, rape, and robbery are wrong, it must also help us with more difficult and complicated issues and questions, such as arise in the health and other professions.

Accountability and responsibility

Being accountable for one's actions or for those of others is to be the one who is "taken to account" or "laid to blame." If something goes wrong and it is my fault, then I am accountable. The third leg of our "overarching stance toward *integrity*," accountability is related to transparency and veracity: If I am accountable for something going wrong, then I am in at least many cases also duty-bound to take public responsibility for it and, in doing so, to tell the truth. That is, mere accountability can be found or determined by others who associate me with the wrongdoing or failure in question. Criminal justice systems exist in part to establish processes for determining accountability or (mere) fault finding. The link to transparency and veracity is why judges sometimes reward or at least reduce the punishment of wrongdoers who confess.

Accountability is related to but distinct from *responsibility*, although in practice the two terms are often used interchangeably. The former is generally applied to events from the time of their occurrence and moving forward, and to mistakes, errors, wrongs, and the like. The latter can also be used for good things that happen ("She is responsible for correcting the dangerous software coding error"), and throughout a process, that is, before any specific event.

Work on the philosophy of accountability dates to Aristotle. What is for the most part uncontroversial is that for a person to be accountable for an action or event, three conditions must be met (Jonas 1984; Noorman 2014). A person must:

- have had some control over the event
- be able to have foreseen the consequences of the event
- be able to act freely

This captures ordinary intuitions about the circumstances under which it makes sense for an individual or, for that matter, aggregates of individuals in laboratories, hospitals, and corporations to be held to account when something goes wrong. That said, we must be careful in a computational environment, that is, one shaped by group efforts, complex products, and millions of lines of computer code. For instance, the first condition above – that one must have had some control over the event – can be difficult to determine because *causation* can be difficult to identify. Our challenge is amplified by the "problem of many hands" (Nissenbaum 1994); and in Chapter 4, it was clear that good practice and attention to quality are important ways to meet the challenges of accountability. It may be said to follow that once the "problem of many hands" is identified and acknowledged, *responsible* entities must make an effort to ensure adequate guidelines and audits for workflow, annotation, attestation, version control, and other standards for writing computer programs and making machines that use them.

This point cannot be overemphasized. In the world of information technology, accountability is a large and rich notion (cf. also Gotterbarn 2001; Johnson 2006). It applies to the manufacture of information processors, the writing of software, and the establishment of processes for information collection, analysis, and use. Because of the complexity of some software, accountability can be difficult to assign, and when we do, it can apply to more than one person, maybe many more. As we saw in Chapter 4, in the discussion of responsible conduct of research, a willingness to be accountable is a mark of integrity. The establishment of processes for error identification and correction itself fosters transparency. This is similar to the best-practice approach to the management of medical errors: Create an environment in which those who make errors are encouraged to disclose them (Hébert et al. 2001).

This approach introduces a tension or conflict between customary views of accountability as emphasizing blameworthiness, sketched just above, and an acknowledgment that assigning blame does not tend to improve quality. Actually, we want both – a kind of accountability without blame so that those who err own their errors but in such a way as to foster openness. Creating such processes is the responsibility of leadership. We have learned from research on medical errors that systems often contribute to, or cause, errors as much or more than individuals. The US Institute of Medicine observed in 1999, "The common initial reaction when an error occurs is to find and blame someone. However, even apparently single events or errors are due most often to the convergence of multiple contributing factors. Blaming an individual does not change these factors and the same error is likely to recur. Preventing errors and improving safety for patients require a systems approach in order to modify the conditions that contribute to errors" (Kohn et al. 1999, 49).

A system of vigorous and transparent oversight, ranging across sloppy coding, human factors management, bug fixes, education, and adherence to standards, is needed to foster a culture of accountability. What has evolved as "accountability training" offered by compliance consulting firms should be adjusted to feature real-world knowledge of the work by professionals being "trained." Fostering accountability in a secretive and proprietary industry is an enormous challenge, but doing so will help produce businesses that do good.[4] Unfortunately, having a business do good is too often different from what is seen as good for business.

Developers, manufacturers, and vendors of electronic health records

The electronic health record industry is unlike any other:

- It makes products that will affect (nearly) all people.
- There is no mechanism for independent oversight or regulation of those products.
- While price and other business considerations form bases for system comparisons, competition is not driven by publicly verifiable measures of safety, quality, efficacy, or efficiency.

Now, if it is correct that health professionals are, by virtue of their education, status, and professional tradition different from other professionals, then those who make their tools must share some of the responsibilities that attach to the practice of nursing and medicine. While all businesses must hew to some ethical standards, those standards will surely vary according as one makes pushpins or pacemakers. In this regard, the electronic health record industry is akin to the pharmaceutical and medical device industries: At the beginning of the line and at the end of the day is a patient.

In traditional industries, the purchaser of a product can reasonably assume that some-one, somewhere, is keeping track of device failures, if not also quality. In Britain and the United States, for example, automobile design, safety, and reporting standards are governed by a constellation of regulatory agencies. If cars are found to have faulty brakes, those cars will eventually be recalled and repaired. Data about brake failures is publicly accessible (transparency),[5] the carmakers sometimes find and report these data (accountability, though required by law), and car buyers can generally rely on these data (veracity). In most industrialized countries, the mechanisms for collecting and analyzing these data are uncontroversial to most car owners, drivers, and passengers. Even the most committed libertarian is unlikely to be sanguine about her grandfather being transported in a vehicle with faulty drums made by the Caveat Emptor Brake Company.

Legal and ethical argumentation

It is commonplace in ethics education to make a bright distinction between ethics and the law. This stance is generally correct: Ethics precedes the law. We must determine if an action is right or wrong before any social system can require or prohibit it. But not the other way round, at least in usual pedagogy: We customarily say that one errs in suggesting that one can learn anything about ethics from the law. But this is a little too quick, and ignores those debates in which legislators and lawyers find themselves in policy arguments and making ethics-like noises in trying to resolve them. Policy debates over abortion, assisted suicide, and access to health care, for instance, can in principle advance our understanding of ethical issues and arguments. So, while it is true that ethics undergirds the law, it is not true that legislators and lawyers are incapable of contributing to ethics debates. For our purposes, a good example comes from contract law. Significantly, the law evolves in concert with society.

Winterbottom v. *Wright*[6] is a hoary classic: an 1842 ruling by the Exchequer of Pleas, the first common law court, dating to the reign of Henry I and dissolved in 1880 after some 800 years. Mr. Wright supplied horse-drawn mail coaches to the Postmaster General and had a contract to keep the coaches in a "fit, proper, safe and secure state and condition." The Postmaster in turn had a contract with one Atkinson to supply horses and coachmen.

Atkinson hired Winterbottom as a driver. But at least one of Wright's coaches was faulty and Winterbottom was thrown from his seat and injured, apparently suffering a lifelong disability. He sued Wright, and lost.

The court held that because Winterbottom had no contract with Wright, he should not be compensated for Wright's negligence. One judge wrote, "There is no privity of contract between these parties; and if the plaintiff can sue, every passenger, or even any person passing along the road, who was injured by the upsetting of the coach, might bring a similar action. Unless we confine the operation of such contracts as this to the parties who entered into them, the most absurd and outrageous consequences, to which I can see no limit, would ensue." Another judge argued, "If we were to hold that the plaintiff could sue in such a case, there is no point at which such actions would stop. The only safe rule is to confine the right to recover to those who enter into the contract: if we go one step beyond that, there is no reason why we should not go fifty. The only real argument in favour of the action is, that this is a case of hardship; but that might have been obviated, if the plaintiff had made himself a party to the contract."

These are utilitarian arguments, concerned about the effect on the courts and society if accountability and responsibility were transitive. If A contracts with B, and B with C, then there would be no end to C suing A anytime something went wrong. The *Winterbottom* court had seen nothing like this case before, and the judges' arguments are not irrational. The integrity of the contract as a means for assigning responsibility was paramount. But this leaves unaddressed any detailed consideration of the legitimacy of a manufacturer's "duty to care" for those downstream who buy or use a faulty product. It was a ruling of the time. The first use of anesthesia during surgery occurs in 1842, when the world's first pilsner beer is brewed, Kropotkin is born, and Stendhal dies. Listen:

> *Winterbottom* v. *Wright* laid down "horse and buggy" law for a "horse and buggy" age – the law that one furnishing chattels to another owes no duty of care to a third party with whom he is not in privity of contract. Yet, even as Winterbottom rode atop the defective mail-coach provided by Wright for the Postmaster-General, the Industrial Revolution was gathering momentum apace; and courts and their law are free, only within limits, to lag behind economic and social change. Law which circumscribed duty within the limits of contract became increasingly incongruous. (Spruill 1941, 551; notes omitted)

Put differently, manufacturers will eventually come to be seen to have duties to those who use their products independently of whether those users had any sort of contract with the manufacturers. This is an example of progress in both ethics and the law. While no philosophers were (apparently) consulted in the 1916 Court of Appeals of New York case of *MacPherson* v. *Buick Motor Co.*, the famous jurist Benjamin N. Cardozo framed the issue as one of duty:

> The defendant is a manufacturer of automobiles. It sold an automobile to a retail dealer. The retail dealer resold to the plaintiff. While the plaintiff was in the car, it suddenly collapsed. He was thrown out and injured. One of the wheels was made of defective wood, and its spokes crumbled into fragments. The wheel was not made by the defendant; it was bought from another manufacturer. There is evidence, however, that its defects could have been discovered by reasonable inspection, and that inspection was omitted. There is no claim that the defendant knew of the defect and willfully concealed it … The charge is one, not of fraud, but of negligence. The question to be determined is whether the defendant owed a duty of care and vigilance to any one but the immediate purchaser.[7]

While the statement of the case is simple, it lays bare the complexities of identifying responsibility and accountability and, hence, sources of product liability. A carmaker might buy wheels from a wheel-maker who buys materials from a steelmaker who obtains iron from an ironmonger ... and so on. And upon this wheel goes a tire, made by a tire-maker who obtains rubber from a rubber-maker who obtains latex from a rubber-tree grower ... . Moreover, these tires and wheels must be designed by someone. Cardozo held that, "If the nature of a thing is such that it is reasonably certain to place life and limb in peril when negligently made, it is then a thing of danger. Its nature gives warning of the consequences to be expected. If to the element of danger there is added knowledge that the thing will be used by persons other than the purchaser, and used without new tests, then, irrespective of contract, the manufacturer of this thing of danger is under a duty to make it carefully."[8]

While it is inexplicit, a *moral* principle underlies his argument. It is this, more or less: When a manufacturer of a device sells it, he is making a kind of promise beyond formal contract to subsequent users that the device will function as intended. This further entails that the manufacturer has a duty to test the device to make good on the promise, thus in principle shrinking the size of the cohort formed by those in the manufacturing chain, or the number of entities responsible under joint and several liability. If a device used in the manner intended causes damage, the manufacturer is both accountable and responsible for the damage. This is in part the foundation of the concept of liability, both moral and legal. One is liable for damages because the damages constitute the breaking of a promise. For poor Winterbottom, the promise ended a step before him; for MacPherson it applied to everyone. Attempts to limit or sidestep this accountability and responsibility are well known in the form of product disclaimers. Some disclaimers are legitimate, some not.

Electronic health record vendor duties

A question that should be confronted by every responsible businessperson goes something like this: Can a disclaimer of *legal* liability absolve me of *moral* responsibility? Relatedly, what kinds of disclaimers are ethically appropriate? What about indemnification and hold-harmless clauses?

It is clear why a business would not want to accept responsibility or be held accountable for a product it has manufactured. Perhaps it has a legitimate fear of being falsely accused. Perhaps its product will be misused. Maybe the product will be altered in ways the company cannot and ought not be responsible for. While such concerns are worthy of consideration, they are not dispositive and should not detract from the brute fact that in some circumstances someone or some organization has (likely) paid for, relied on, and been injured by a product. Sorting out who is at fault might very well be complicated, but this is why civil society has mechanisms for doing just that. That a product manufacturer might want to foreclose on all liability in advance – even with a reason – by an initial declaration of nonresponsibility is at least sometimes to put the interests of the manufacturer ahead of the user. Now, this might very well be innocuous for many things, but there is broad and uncontroversial agreement that it should not be applied to pharmaceutical or medical products – drugs and devices intended for use in or for a sick human or animal.

There are several reasons for this, and they point to the utility of ethics in the development of public policy. One way to begin is to identify and rank or order the things we value.

If it turns out that we generally value free speech, say, more than public tranquility, for instance, then it makes sense to permit offensive speech at the expense of amity. What is significant is that the two values need not always be in conflict – we just need to be prepared to assign one priority when they are. Here is another example: We value the right to refuse medical interventions, but we also value not contracting polio, so the desire to refuse polio vaccination is legitimately opposed when someone actually tries to invoke a right rarely challenged at other times. We value human safety and life more than the unfettered expression of entrepreneurial genius – and so we have in the modern era a history of regulating biomedical research, of laws governing the marketing and sale of drugs, of regulations applied to drug and device manufacture, and of oversight in the food, auto- motive, aeronautic, and medical industries.

The challenge we face is this: How can legitimate business interests be protected, innovation be stimulated, and health and safety be secured – simultaneously – in and for the multibillion-dollar international electronic health record industry, alleged a little earlier to be unique because of its scope, freedom from regulation, and absence of criteria- or evidence-based competition? One important critique of the industry reported that EHR vendors have created and insist on contracts that enable them to "enjoy a contractual and legal structure that renders them virtually liability free – 'hold harmless' is the term of art – even when their proprietary products may be implicated in adverse events involving patients" (Koppel and Kreda 2009, 1276).

The doctrine that guides such a contractual provision is not implausible. Physicians and nurses use electronic health records for decision support, patient data retrieval, and various kinds of calculations. If something were to go wrong with the system, then it makes some sense for the user, already competent in medicine or nursing, to be able to detect and correct the malfunction. That idea, at least, is what shapes the theory underlying the "learned intermediary" doctrine, introduced in Chapter 2. Invented in the United States in the mid-twentieth century,[9] it initially pertained to product liability as applied to prescription drugs, is the central idea being that a manufacturer's purported duty to warn of side-effects can be discharged by informing physicians about drug risks. Then, if anything goes wrong, it is the physicians' fault. A pharmaceutical company can argue that it does not practice medicine, or know individual patients' medical histories, and therefore that the locus of responsibility should lie with those who do. The doctrine invites many exceptions, not least in a world in which market share hunger drives drug and device companies to reach out directly to patients. Direct-to-consumer advertising, a bad idea in any civil society, undermines the role of physician as learned and as an intermediary.[10] The rise and apparent commercial success of direct-to-consumer advertising implies that the pharmaceutical industry was willing to wager that such advertising would increase sales in an amount greater than would be lost in court without the learned intermediary doctrine to prophylax against faulty products.

The doctrine solved a responsibility-assignment problem for the courts, albeit in an industry long regulated and whose intellectual property is protected by patent and other intellectual property law. The EHR industry enjoys no regulation. Moreover, even the most junior member of the Research Ethics Committee or Institutional Review Board is privy to study protocols laying out drugs' chemical structure and hypothesized mechanism of action, as well as the detailed research plan for testing the drug in humans. The electronic health record industry's proprietary information is not available for any similar quasi-public scrutiny. (It is curious that physicians have not protested that the doctrine actually makes increasingly less sense in a world in which no amount of medical expertise can parse a pharmacopeia bloated with me-too drugs and of nontrivial genomic and environmental variation among patients.)

All this is to say that the application of the learned intermediary doctrine to health information technology (HIT), including electronic health record and decision support systems, is a stratagem in futile search of ethical warrant. This claim requires elaboration.

After the publication of Koppel and Kreda's watershed critique, the Board of Directors of AMIA (formerly the American Medical Informatics Association), the leading professional organization in health informatics, established a task force and commissioned a report, "Challenges in ethics, safety, best practices, and oversight regarding HIT vendors, their customers, and patients: a report of an AMIA special task force" (Goodman et al. 2011). The task force included representatives from the HIT/EHR industry and a number of academics, including one of the authors of the publication that triggered the assignment. The report had two overarching findings, distilled and simplified here: The industry should be able to realize a return on investment, enjoy profits, and experience growth; *and* it should not do so by using contract language to force health care institutions to assume all liability come what may or to restrain trade or communication related to system performance.

The last finding was motivated by the allegation that commercial contract language includes not only hold-harmless clauses but also nondisclosure language that compels system users not to communicate about systems' "problematic, even disastrous, software faults. Even though enforced nonsharing of software problems is an industry norm, it is anathema to improving care, to HIT, and to evidence-based medicine" (Koppel and Kreda 2009, 1277). (It is important to note that it is also difficult to obtain copies of EHR contracts, and that confirmation of the existence of offensive provisions is correspondingly challenging. This is an area deserving of more and deeper scrutiny.) In greater detail, these are among the task force's recommendations:

> Contracts should not contain language that prevents system users, including clinicians and others, from using their best judgment about what actions are necessary to protect patient safety. This includes freedom to disclose system errors or flaws, whether introduced or caused by the vendor, the client, or any other third party. Disclosures made in good faith should not constitute violations of HIT contracts. This recommendation neither entails nor requires the disclosure of trade secrets or intellectual property ...
>
> Because vendors and their customers share responsibility for patient safety, contract provisions should not attempt to circumvent fault and should recognize that both vendors and purchasers share responsibility for successful implementation. For example, vendors should not be absolved from harm resulting from system defects, poor design or usability, or hard-to-detect errors. Similarly, purchasers should not be absolved from harm resulting from inadequate training and education, inadequate resourcing, customization, or inappropriate use ...
>
> Contracts should require that system defects, software deficiencies, and implementation practices that threaten patient safety should be reported, and information about them be made available to others, as appropriate ...   (Goodman et al. 2011, 78–79)

These and other recommendations were intended to be uncontroversial. That is, with agreement that (i) transparency is an elemental and non-negotiable business value and

(ii) businesses making products used in health care have the additional duty to embrace at least a minimum level of patient-centeredness, then, it is not clear how or why someone would want to disagree – unless she wanted or needed recourse to something like a learned intermediary rule to provide liability insulation. Recall that poor Mr. Winterbottom fell off his defective mail coach in the wrong century. Had he been thrown from an equally faulty automobile, he would have been able to hold the manufacturer to account and, indeed, before that, would have drawn some comfort in knowing that the instruments of civil society were being used to require that automobile manufacturers ensured that their vehicles were safe in the first place.

Cast in this way, the quest for learned intermediaries – experts who somehow do not merely practice medicine but also are expert in computer programming, pharmacology, organic chemistry, and the genetics of personalized medicine – emerges as a stretch, a gambit, a stratagem not to apportion responsibility accurately and fairly, but to shirk it. Indeed, even the perfect learned intermediary does not order patients to take medicines; her job is to counsel and recommend. If a patient who is mindful of the risks of taking a government-regulated drug does so and is harmed, then, however, does it make sense to say the physician is responsible and to hold her accountable? Observe that the ethical and legal rules for valid or informed consent in clinical practice and biomedical research require that patients or subjects be informed about risks, potential benefits, and alternatives to a particular treatment or research intervention, and that the patient/subject make a voluntary decision, that is, one free of undue influence, inappropriate pressure, or coercion. If an informed patient/subject makes a voluntary choice to take a drug – believing that the potential benefits are worth the risks as disclosed – then we say that while the patient might later be *harmed*, he was not *wronged*. Absent any separate but related wrongdoing by the drug or device manufacturer, it would not be fair to the manufacturer to hold it accountable.

Toward a patient-centered health information technology industry

The idea that electronic health records should be patient centered is not new, at least in its stipulation. For the most part, however, it has been an approach emphasizing clinical or home-based encounters. So it has been suggested that electronic health records should, for instance, not impede clinician–patient communication (Ventres and Frankel 2010), can contribute to medication reconciliation (Greenwald et al. 2010), and are essential for patient care in electronic medical homes (Bates and Bitton 2010; Meyers et al. 2010). The thesis here is different. It is not that electronic health records can contribute to better patient care; it is that corporations that make these systems have a duty to patients similar to the duties of the clinicians who use the systems. This is a claim that for-profit corporations have duties to their customers' patients' well-being. The discharge of that duty requires, at a minimum, adequate privacy and confidentiality provisions, interoperability, evidence-based decision support, and so on. It also means assumption of responsibility for the deliverable, in the same way that no credible physician would attempt to create a process under which she would treat a patient only if the patient agreed in advance to indemnify and hold the physician harmless for bad outcomes.

It was earlier hypothesized that "No developer or seller of electronic health records would ever publicly confess that, 'Our business plan is to acquire vast personal and corporate wealth based on the misfortunes of sick people.' " The point was a kind of moral *reductio ad absurdum* – not a stepwise argument, but a cut-to-the-chase observation based on the idea that healers and those who make their tools have as legitimate missions the reduction of suffering and the lengthening of life, and to deny that mission leads to absurdity. No little time was then spent on enlarging and celebrating the importance of transparency, veracity, and responsibility/accountability. But suppose that some health care professional were perfectly transparent, a model of veracity, and an unflinching accepter of responsibility and accountability – but cared not a whit for patients. He says, "I'm OK with transparency, veracity, and accountability – but I am not a social service agency, and do not give a rip about sick people as such. If they suffer and die, they suffer and die. How did that become my responsibility?"

There are several responses to this. They touch on the foundations of ethics in health care. We can enumerate several, but will stop at three. First, healers are, by virtue of their education and, traditionally and historically, at least, their motivation, therefore, obligated, as a matter of professionalism and personal integrity or character, to be self-effacing and to promote patient interests ahead of their own. This, we teach our medical and nursing students, is the ethos and history of the health professional; if you do not like it, get another job. Second, if one can help, then one ought to help. In one simple and powerful formulation, the philosopher Peter Singer has us imagine a child who has fallen into a shallow pond and is drowning. I could easily wade in and save him, except that doing so would make my clothes muddy. If we agree the loss of a life is worse than the loss of a shoe, I must rescue the child (Singer 1972).[11] Moreover, if I have special training in lifesaving, then my duties increase correspondingly. Indeed, if anyone has special training to save lives, then one must save lives – everything else pales in significance. Third, what goes around comes around. If it is true that I would prefer a physician who put my interests ahead of hers, then on pain of hypocrisy would I adopt a different course if I were a physician.

Cast informally, these three mini-arguments for patient-centeredness also rely on three core systems or theories in moral philosophy, namely, virtue ethics, Utilitarianism, and deontology. They all give the same answer. The goal here is not to defend a patient-centric approach for clinicians but rather to underscore how this value can be applied to HIT and EHR vendors (and, by extension, anyone who makes tools for doctors and nurses). As given above, we could rely on a *reductio* argument, but it might be preferable to state the case positively. Indeed, this positive argument has been threaded throughout this chapter, and we can summarize it now:

HIT and EHR vendors should be patient-centered on analogy with clinicians and hospitals because, as discussed above:

- "… they are [or soon will become] necessary to human health and survival, [and therefore] owe the world the same thing as a physician or nurse – at least some selflessness."
- "… patients are not analogous to investors, shareholders, customers or any such thing."
- "… the EHR industry is akin to the pharmaceutical and medical device industries: At the beginning of the line and at the end of the day is a patient."

Therefore, EHR vendors themselves have a duty to this professional brand of patient-centeredness.

In the same way the libertarian Hayek saw no contradiction in safety-net hospitals, there is none to be found here in concluding that even a for-profit business owes something large and of ancient provenance to sick people. Even a fiduciary duty to investors, shareholders, and speculators does not permit, let alone require, neglecting patient safety. More importantly, imagine an EHR industry in which firms competed on the basis of price, adherence to standards, and quality, where all these were assessed based on measurable public criteria – just like automobile manufacturers, airplane builders, and medical device makers. To the extent that these criteria reduce harm, we may regard those who hew to them as having some commitment to those for whom these things were made. At ground, remember, for such a system to be regarded as driver-, passenger- or patient-centered, those purporting to make the commitment must also embrace the values of transparency, veracity, and responsibility/accountability. Surely there is no market pressure strong enough to frustrate or impede such an embrace. Equally certainly, no credible EHR maker would desire anything else, and surely none would publicly admit to waiting until required by law for its consummation.

Regulation of the health information technology industry

If ever there were a good example of the relationship between ethics and public policy – and of the utility of the former in shaping the latter – it is the question whether electronic health records should be regulated. That is actually just the first of five questions, the answers to which are needed to support a thoughtful and balanced policy: Should the industry be regulated? If so, by whom or what? Then, what precisely is to be regulated? To what extent? Moreover, with what assessment and evaluation tools? While a worthy project, it is also quite large. Here is an overview of what such a project might look like in terms of the ethical issues raised in debates over the regulation of electronic health records.

Historically, most ethico-policy debates are won or lost (or, rather, should be won or lost) according as one side presents better evidence of prevention or reduction of harms and wrongs or maximization of goods than the other. For the utilitarian, of course, there are no wrongs other than harms: Good and bad, right and wrong, blameworthy and praiseworthy are a function of harms, goods, and other consequences. Under a rule- or rights-based moral theory, contrarily, individuals and perhaps groups have various legitimate (claims to) entitlements. It is very difficult to identify these entitlements, especially in a computational world. Even a "right to privacy," as we saw in Chapter 3, and will discuss again in Chapter 8, is not absolute and may sometimes be abridged to prevent harms or to maximize benefits to others.[12]

The regulation of drugs and medical devices is fundamentally utilitarian. The deceptively promoted and dangerous "patent medicines" of the nineteenth and early twentieth centuries led to widespread regulation in many countries. (For a trip down this toxic memory lane, see the American Medical Association's *Nostrums and Quackery* 1910.) While there is no credible or serious opposition to the policy that drugs and devices should be regulated, considerable debate attaches to the question whether government regulation should include electronic health records and their components. There are two main arguments against regulation. One turns on the regulatory question whether electronic health records are medical devices of the sort for which there is, in the United States, ample precedent for Food and Drug Administration (FDA) regulation:

The term "device" ... means an instrument, apparatus, implement, machine, contrivance, implant, in vitro reagent, or other similar or related article, including any component, part, or accessory, which is –

(1) recognized in the official National Formulary, or the United States Pharmacopeia, or any supplement to them,

(2) intended for use in the diagnosis of disease or other conditions, or in the cure, mitigation, treatment, or prevention of disease, in man or other animals, or

(3) intended to affect the structure or any function of the body of man or other animals, and which does not achieve its primary intended purposes through chemical action within or on the body of man or other animals and which is not dependent upon being metabolized for the achievement of its primary intended purposes.[13]

If an electronic health record is a Class III device, then it can be regulated as such. As a result, no little effort has gone into parsing the definition, and reasonable people continue to disagree. The Institute of Medicine's 2012 report, *Health IT and Patient Safety: Building Safer Systems for Better Care*, was agnostic on the issue, saying, "FDA has chosen to not exercise regulatory authority over EHRs, and controversy exists over whether some health IT products such as EHRs should be considered medical devices"[14] (but see Cook 2012 for an argument that systems should be regulated as such). The institute recommends that the Secretary of Health and Human Services "should monitor and publicly report on the progress of health IT safety ... If progress toward safety and reliability is not sufficient as determined by the Secretary, the Secretary should direct FDA to exercise all available authorities to regulate EHRs, health information exchanges, and PHRs ... [the Secretary] should immediately direct FDA to begin developing the necessary framework for regulation. Such a framework should be in place if and when the Secretary decides the state of health IT safety requires FDA regulation" (Institute of Medicine 2012, 13).[15]

The second argument against regulation is it will stifle innovation. Both the FDA and Britain's Medicines and Healthcare products Regulatory Agency (MHRA) are familiar with the argument (cf. Cohen 2013; Sorenson and Drummond 2014). To be sure, the argument from innovation embeds an empirical claim, although it is not clear how it would be tested. There are several possible responses to the argument:

Good show – ensure there is no government regulation of electronic health records lest it have a chilling effect on innovation.

Nonsense – there is no evidence or other reason to support the chilling-effect-on-innovation allegation, and electronic records are already documented to pose safety risks in at least some circumstances.

Are you serious? – electronic records are not very good and lack innovation in the first place, and any lack of innovation is due to no fault of government regulators. Regulation might even spur innovation if done rightly. Other regulated industries seem somehow to innovate.

We are unlikely – and, indeed, for our purposes, do not need – to resolve this issue here.[16] We would not be amiss, however, in urging continued assessment of all forms of oversight, credentialing, and regulation. For instance, it is not clear that adequate attention has been devoted to the idea (Miller and Gardner 1997a, 1997b) that some health software might be evaluated by "autonomous software oversight committees" analogous to research ethics committees or the institutional review boards that are trusted with protection of human subjects.

One of the arguments for this conclusion lies in the FDA's perpetual underfunding, that is, lack of resources. At the seam between ethics and policy, one way to get the policies one wants without the ethics one needs is to ensure that otherwise standard and uncontroversial government mechanisms for regulation do not have enough money to do their jobs.

Shared responsibilities

In early 2015, an extraordinary group of 35 US medical societies, led by the American Medical Association, asked the Office of the National Coordinator for Health Information Technology to decouple EHR certification from the meaningful use program, in part because of concerns that the process is disconnected from actual system performance and that the systems continue to lack interoperability (Hirsch 2015). Specifically:

> We believe there is an urgent need to change the current certification program to better align end-to-end testing to focus on EHR usability, interoperability, and safety. We understand from discussions with the Office of the National Coordinator for Health Information Technology (ONC) that there is an interest in improving the current certification program. For the reasons outlined in detail below, we strongly recommend the following changes to EHR certification:
>
> 1. *Decouple EHR certification from the Meaningful Use program;*
> 2. *Re-consider alternative software testing methods;*
> 3. *Establish greater transparency and uniformity on [user centered design] testing and process results;*
> 4. *Incorporate exception handling into EHR certification;*
> 5. *Develop [consolidated clinical document architecture] guidance and tests to support exchange;*
> 6. *Seek further stakeholder feedback; and*
> 7. *Increase education on EHR implementation.*[17]

What this seems to illustrate is that there is quite enough responsibility and accountability to go around. What the Institute of Medicine called a "shared responsibility for improving health IT safety" (2012, 6ff.) makes clear that even careful, non-innovation-stifling regulation does not relieve all stakeholders of duties to contribute to the project. This recapitulates the point made in Chapter 1, as we began stating simple if not obvious "ethical obligations" ranging across stakeholders. The angry Bernard Shaw, who helped begin this discussion, gets the last word: "We are made wise not by the recollection of our past, but by the responsibility for our future."

Notes

1. This is also partly why some commercial considerations will always be intrusions, and therefore should not be permitted. Imagine a hospital or system vendor advancing the idea of selling pharmaceutical advertising to appear on electronic health record screens, like ads on a Web page; or that certain diagnoses or diagnostic codes, when entered, would trigger advertisements for drugs to treat that which was diagnosed; and that the entire project would be touted as a form of "sponsored decision support."

2. There is a large and interesting debate about how much and what ought to be disclosed during the consent process. One of the most challenging questions concerns whether to reveal complex data regarding volume outcome studies, which tend to find that individuals and hospitals with higher volumes tend to have better results. It is worth noting that such studies can be conducted in real time and updated periodically; and patients themselves can in principle consult published outcomes; in the future they might very well be able to use the Web to conduct their own comparisons. Should you tell your patient, "I'm OK at this, but the evidence shows that you are likely to have a better result if you went to the hospital across town"...? See Stell 2014 for a good review, but the wrong conclusion.

3. The philosophical literature on truth, truthlikeness, verisimilitude, and so on is large, complex, and unlikely to be appreciated casually. Scholars in the philosophy of science are mainly concerned with the role of truth in the sciences; those in the philosophy of language focus on its role in speech and logic; and scientific language itself is a locus of many analyses. A reliable source of introductions to standard issues in philosophy is *The Stanford Encyclopedia of Philosophy* (http://plato.stanford.edu/); and on this topic Glanzberg 2014.

4. "Artificial agents" themselves might have moral obligations. This was anticipated long before there were useful robots:

   1—A robot may not injure a human being, or, through inaction, allow a human being to come to harm.

   2—A robot must obey the orders given it by human beings except where such orders would conflict with the First Law.

   3—A robot must protect its own existence as long as such protection does not conflict with the First or Second Law.

   The Three Laws of Robotics, *Handbook of Robotics*, 56th Edition, 2058 A.D.   (Asimov 1950)

   The "morality of artificial agents" is given a nice analysis by Luciano Floridi (2013) and criticized as "infeasible" by Hew (2014); cf. Nissenbaum (1994). The Illinois Institute of Technology philosopher John Snapper (1998) suggested that there were good utilitarian grounds – future patients would be better served – by assigning responsibility to intelligent machines themselves. In brief, if there is reason to believe computers will improve health care, and if they are so complex as to make it unfair to assign accountability to the manufacturer, then we should "encourage the use of good technology by absolving the clinician of some accountability" (p. 54). The best way to do that is to include the intelligent machine in the web of accountability. In an extended personal communication, quoted and edited with permission, Snapper writes:

   I see several forces at play in the evolution of a modern theory of responsibility. For instance, (a) philosophers commenting on philosophers tend to deepen the notion of responsibility and make it more complex. So Kant's views are deepened through Schopenhauer's commentaries and Schopenhauer's views are deepened through Nietzsche's commentaries. This also holds when we reach back for inspiration to the classics. When Nussbaum draws on Aristotle for inspiration, she adds complexity and sophistication to Rawls' concept of responsibility. (b) Shifts in institutional practices push responsibility in new directions, demanding philosophical responses. When the U.S. Federal Reserve System or central bank imposes rules or when we impose rules on the Fed, we change the way we assess responsibility of lenders and borrowers. Every tweak to the criminal law, every decision on torts, leads to reconsiderations and new understandings of behavioral responsibility within jurisdictions. (c) And of particular interest, there are the consequences of shifts in technology. I love to watch how philosophers comment on the shifts. When surgery is practiced in teams rather than by individual doctors, when schizophrenia is identified with physiological pathologies, when the fetus can be diagnosed with problems, then the philosophy community jumps in with revisions to the concept of responsibility, helping it evolve to confront new issues.

   All this pushes a pair of comments on Darwin's conception of the evolution of morality. Few of us read *The Descent of Man* with any care today. But if you do, you will see that the central problem in the book is the evolution of an animal that acts with true morality. Unlike modern evolutionists, Darwin sets the human higher in the animal kingdom than the other animals. We have evolved further than the crow and the chimp. And the primary mark of that higher status is true morality and benevolence. The last sentence of the book remarks on "man with all his noble qualities, with sympathy that extends to the most debased, with benevolence which extends not only to other men but to the humblest living creature ..." It is the evolution of that benevolence which is the central story of the book. Darwin has a particularly hard time explaining the evolution of morality, given the fierceness of natural selection that at some level selects through extinction.

   Darwin explains the evolution of "social instincts" with stories about group selection (or what we now call "kinship selection"). A herd of wolves that shares meat has an advantage on a herd of selfish wolves. Darwin will use such observations to explain the evolution of social cooperation, maternal love, and related behaviors which are exhibited by the "lower" animals. What few readers notice, however, is that Darwin partly abandons that story for what he sees as the final steps in human evolution of benevolence. After all, stories about group evolution cannot explain why a human would be sympathetic to someone from a distant tribe or race, and certainly not why we should care to save the whales. Sometimes Darwin meets the challenge with Lamarckian stories about the learned acceptance of responsibility. But I think that the central argument is actually quite Kantian. The argument is that humans have evolved separately both social instincts and intellectual skills. Applying our newly evolved intellect to an understanding of our newly evolved social instincts, we humans can figure out why the social instincts are morally correct. In this way we arrive at true morality, based in an intellectual understanding of humane behavior. So for Darwin, true ethics is ultimately based in something vaguely like Kantian intellection of duty.

5. In the United States, for instance, the National Highway Traffic Safety Administration maintains a comprehensive Web site (www.nhtsa.gov) and searchable databases to help car owners learn about vehicle safety and to search for information on specific defects.

6. *Winterbottom* v. *Wright*, 10 M&W 109; 152 ER 402 (1842).

7. *MacPherson* v. *Buick Motor Co.*, 217 N.Y. 382, 111 N.E. 1050 (1916).

8. He concludes:

    We think the defendant was not absolved from a duty of inspection because it bought the wheels from a reputable manufacturer. It was not merely a dealer in automobiles. It was a manufacturer of automobiles. It was responsible for the finished product. It was not at liberty to put the finished product on the market without subjecting the component parts to ordinary and simple tests *(Richmond & Danville R. R. Co.* v. *Elliott,* 149 U.S. 266, 272). Under the charge of the trial judge nothing more was required of it. The obligation to inspect must vary with the nature of the thing to be inspected. The more probable the danger, the greater the need of caution ... Both by its relation to the work and by the nature of its business, [the manufacturer] is charged with a stricter duty.

    Cardozo cites *Winterbottom* and notes apparently contradictory rulings in other English courts. But it is clear he thinks the Winterbottom court erred: "There is nothing anomalous in a rule which imposes upon A, who has contracted with B, a duty to C and D and others according as he knows or does not know that the subject-matter of the contract is intended for their use."

    The issues of privity and third-party rights remain sources of scholarship and policy. Britain's Law Commission produced a useful international review in 1996 (Law Commission 1996). Cf. Palmer (1983, 1992).

9. *Marcus* v. *Specific Pharmaceuticals, Inc.*, 77 N.Y.S.2d 508 (App. Div. 1948). The term "learned intermediary" is apparently first used in *Sterling Drug* v. *Cornish*, 370 F.2d 82, 85 (8th Cir. 1966).

10. The first exception to the doctrine is *Perez* v. *Wyeth Labs*, 161 N.J. 1, 24 (1999).

11. Singer's goal was to establish and defend an account of our duties to respond to suffering anywhere, in part by contributions to collective efforts. His famous article was published during the famine in the province of East Bengal, later East Pakistan, preceding the creation of Bangladesh. He wrote:

    if it is in our power to prevent something bad from happening, without thereby sacrificing anything of comparable moral importance, we ought, morally, to do it. By "without sacrificing anything of comparable moral importance" I mean without causing anything else comparably bad to happen, or doing something that is wrong in itself, or failing to promote some moral good, comparable in significance to the bad thing that we can prevent. This principle seems almost as uncontroversial as the last one. It requires us only to prevent what is bad, and to promote what is good, and it requires this of us only when we can do it without sacrificing anything that is, from the moral point of view, comparably important. (Singer 1972, 231)

12. Remember John Stuart Mill:

    And it seems to me that in consequence of the absence of rule or principle, one side is at present as often wrong as the other: the interference of government is, with about equal frequency, improperly invoked and improperly condemned ... the sole end for which mankind are warranted, individually or collectively, in interfering with the liberty of action of any of their number, is self-protection. That the only purpose for which power can be rightfully exercised over any member of a civilized community, against his will, is to prevent harm to others. (Mill 1956, 12–13)

13. Federal Food, Drug, and Cosmetic Act, 21 U.S.C. § 321 SEC. 201, 2006–2010.

14. More fully:

The committee was of mixed opinion on how FDA regulation would impact the pace of innovation by industry but identified several areas of concern regarding immediate FDA regulation. The current FDA framework is oriented toward conventional, out-of-the-box, turnkey devices. However, health IT has multiple different characteristics, suggesting that a more flexible regulatory framework will be needed in this area to achieve the goals of product quality and safety without unduly constraining market innovation. For example, as a software-based product, health IT has a product life cycle very different from that of conventional technologies. These products exhibit great diversity in features, functions, and scope of intended and actual use, which tend to evolve over the life of the product. Taking a phased, risk-based approach can help address this concern. FDA has chosen to not exercise regulatory authority over EHRs, and controversy exists over whether some health IT products such as EHRs should be considered medical devices. If the Secretary deems it necessary for FDA to regulate EHRs and other currently nonregulated health IT products, clear determinations will need to be made about whether all health IT products classify as medical devices for the purposes of regulation. If FDA regulation is deemed necessary, FDA will need to commit sufficient resources and add capacity and expertise to be effective. (Institute of Medicine 2012, 12)

15. The FDA's current thinking appears to be laid out in the document "Medical Device Accessories: Defining Accessories and Classification Pathway for New Accessory Types: Draft Guidance for Industry and Food and Drug Administration Staff," available at www.fda.gov/downloads/MedicalDevices/DeviceRegulationand Guidance/GuidanceDocuments/UCM429672.pdf?source=govdelivery&utm_medium=email&utm_source=govdelivery.

Cf. the FDA's decision to regulate some mobile health devices, e.g., phones as a component of an electrocardiogram device or which can measure blood glucose: www.fda.gov/MedicalDevices/Productsand MedicalProcedures/ConnectedHealth/MobileMedicalApplications/ucm255978.htm.

16. For a commentary on the "ethics of regulation" in another health context, see De Ville (1999).

17. Original emphasis, available at http://mb.cision.com/Public/373/9710840/9053557230dbb768.pdf.

Chapter 7

Digital health
Ubiquitous, virtual, remote, robotic

That the Internet has changed everything has become a commonplace observation. That it expands and perhaps alters the ethical challenges faced by clinicians, corporations, and institutions remains a source of exciting empirical and ethical inquiry. Social networking, consumer health informatics, mobile health, and remote care deserve comprehensive research programs. The identification of salient issues is the first step. Their resolution, when possible, will be based on traditional methods and criteria, as well as the results of those research efforts. When a resolution is not yet possible, one option is to embrace a modicum of skepticism. This is not necessarily to signal a negative stance. It is, rather, to make clear that after a long tradition of laying on of hands, we should accept alterations in health practice only with good – perhaps really good – reasons.

Information versus learning

In a breathtakingly short time, ordinary people have acquired the ability to access and contribute to the world's store of health information. It is not yet clear if that is good or not. There are a great many people and that is a great deal of information, and one might plausibly inquire whether life is better for it and, indeed, how we would know. Herbert A. Simon, the 1978 Nobel laureate in economics, who also worked in psychology, the philosophy of science, and computer science (and may be said to be the only philosopher since Sartre to win a Nobel Prize; Sartre refused to accept his in 1964), was skeptical, or at least worried:

> in an information-rich world, the wealth of information means a dearth of something else: a scarcity of whatever it is that information consumes. What information consumes is rather obvious: it consumes the attention of its recipients. Hence a wealth of information creates a poverty of attention and a need to allocate that attention efficiently among the overabundance of information sources that might consume it.   (Simon 1971, 40–1)

This is not merely a complaint about new opportunities for crypto-hypochondriacs to fool around too much online. It is, rather, a challenge that grips at the core of the Information Age. We use the term "bandwidth" to describe how much data can be transmitted by a medium. Simon is concerned about *cognitive bandwidth*, or our ability to get at, make sense of, or, most broadly and metaphorically, metabolize large volumes of information. Put differently, information in all its great volume exacts a price. It is true that (a) Staphylococcus aureus protein A has the UniProt identifier P38507, (b) *S. aureus* is Gram positive, (c) Patient X has methicillin-resistant *Staphylococcus aureus* (MRSA), and (d) germs cause disease. All of this and much more is easily available on the World Wide

Web, as data, information, or knowledge, but its utility is differential, depending on one's role, needs, and cognitive bandwidth. Saul Bellow, the novelist and another Nobelist, was mostly concerned with journalism when he wrote, "We are informed about everything. We know nothing" (Bellow 1977); but we can take the point.

If health information is to be of real use – to improve health, for instance – then we must figure out how best to add to it and use it. This, in turn, requires an exploration of some of the ways we have decoupled health care from what is customarily called the "point of care." In principle and increasingly, a point of care can be anywhere. Along the way, a variety of ethical issues comes into focus and are related to the Internet and World Wide Web, including consumer health informatics, mobile health, personal health records, mobile health and wearable devices, medical homes and ubiquitous monitoring, and robots and digital companions.

The Internet, Web, and consumer health informatics

As the Internet, a network, and the World Wide Web, an information exchange medium atop it, evolved, they quickly embraced health care. Imagine being able to look up information and get advice – reliable information and good advice – quickly and easily, or to communicate rapidly and securely with a physician or nurse while at home. Health care at a distance was and remains a rich source of ethical issues for patients, clinicians, institutions, and civil society itself. While some of these issues are integral to specific media, some are not. That is, some ethical issues depend on a medium and some do not; moreover, in some cases, it is either not clear or the answer is "a little of both." If one can commit a murder or break into a house with a hammer, it does not follow that we need to develop a curriculum and require all hammer owners to attend a workshop in Hammer Ethics. Likewise guitars, prosthetic legs, or crucifixes, all of which have been used to kill people.

Some uses of information and communication technology raise ethical issues in ways perfectly parallel to that of other media. So, for instance, there is nothing of special ethical significance about using a Web site to trick people into sending money for bogus unguents for arthritis, weight loss, or breast enlargement – nothing, that is, about the Web that makes it worse than using the television, telephone, or matchbook cover for the same purposes. It is wrong to do such things, but such wrongness is independent of the medium.

That said, there is something to be said for the idea that by its sheer magnitude, there is something special about health on the Web. What the World Health Organization calls "The Health Internet" is simultaneously the largest health library in the history of civilization, the largest source of advice, and the largest number of connections among patients and between patients and caregivers. Where a decade and a half ago our concerns emphasized accuracy, quality, and the marketplace (Anderson and Goodman 2002; Cline and Haynes 2001), we have grown to occupy ourselves with an ubiquitous source of information and communication that shapes behavior, affects the health of populations, and fundamentally changes the way we think of illness management (cf. Abaidoo and Larweh 2014).

We should assume for the sake of discussion that health-related Web sites hew to values we have emphasized throughout the book, and especially in Chapters 4 and 6, namely transparency, veracity, and accountability/responsibility, which are the values needed to establish integrity and foster trust. What, thereafter, should attract our attention? Consider the following:

- 81% of US adults use the Internet; 72% of those say they have "looked online for health information in the past year."
- 35% of those, called "online diagnosers," "have gone online to figure out what they or someone else might have."
- Of those, 46% reported they needed to see a physician.
- 38% took care of it at home.
- 11% said it was either "both or in-between" professional attention and home care.
- 41% said a medical professional confirmed their "diagnosis," and, of the rest, some either did not get a professional opinion (35%), received one that disagreed (18%), or had an "inconclusive" encounter (1%).
- Females, whites, the affluent, and the young were more likely to try to find a diagnosis. (Fox and Duggan 2013, 6; cf. Bundorf et al. 2006; McDaid and Park 2011. It should be emphasized that these and subsequent sources have surveyed different cohorts at different times, and therefore statistics here and following do not admit of congruent, across-the-board comparisons. Nevertheless, there is general agreement among sources. For historical perspective, see Baker et al. 2003.)
- Of all topics, the 10 most searched-for were flu, cold, labor, diarrhea, balance, diet, back pain, allergies, rash, lupus (Fox 2013).

In Britain, 43% of all adults looked for health information online; users were slightly older than those in the United States, but with similar gender ratios (Office for National Statistics 2013); 41% of Canadian adults consult sites devoted to specific diseases, issues, or products (CBC 2011); in France, 48% of young adults used the Internet for medical and health purposes (Beck et al. 2014).

This is to say that the Internet has both expanded and changed the way people try to manage their well-being. While far too much commentary about health online tends toward hyperbole or overstatement, at this granularity it might be permissible: The Internet has changed everything. Two to three generations ago, medical libraries were remote, inaccessible, or off limits to most people. Someone who wanted to learn about a malady could try to read up on it in an encyclopedia or public library reference; it was generally a frustrating and unilluminating experience. The very idea that a layperson might type a simple list of symptoms into a browser's "search" field and actually learn something was unthinkable.[1]

That browser might be on a telephone or tablet. The utility of such a rough-and-ready source of health information remains to be assessed; however, its scope does not. That is, the growth of mobile-health accessories is rapid and wide, and, in some contexts, of greatest use to those perhaps to be regarded most vulnerable by virtue of their chronic maladies and barriers to traditional health care (Bundorf et al. 2006). In emerging economies (are all patients in such regions vulnerable?), there is often no alternative. With graphic presentations that might strike some as lurid, they, nevertheless, can be the best and only access to health care information.[2] What this might mean is that any reliable ethics targeting system will pick out different issues according as socioeconomic status varies.

Consider the common observation, often *qua* clinician complaint, that patients too often go online and begin to form views about their symptoms before seeking professional attention; worse, they sometime arrive at their appointments knowing more about something than the nurse or physician. This is arguably more a problem with control than content. We have spent generations teaching medical and nursing students that good communication, improved health literacy, and patient engagement are valuable compo-nents of successful clinical relationships. So there should really be more to celebrate than disdain when a patient shows up for her appointment with a sheaf of pages printed (or links saved) from the Web. Use the occasion as a teaching moment about the differential reliability of Web sites. It is when a patient who needs professional attention stumbles about the Web but then fails to get that attention that we must worry.

Mobile health by necessity or by convenience?

First, as above, assume as an ethical baseline that Web sites and mobile applications are designed to, and actually do, reflect the core values of transparency, veracity, and accountability.

Second, we should continuously document effectiveness in salient populations. There is a growing body of data suggesting that mobile tools can improve health in both low- and high-income countries. Is this because the new technology is filling preexisting gaps in the health care spectrum or because it is improving care, or outcomes, atop an acceptably high standard?

Third, decide among improving the basic health care infrastructure, broadening collec-tive reliance on the Internet and mobile health care, or both.

The mobile- and e-health literatures are growing rapidly, with exciting but inconclusive evidence that information technology is a powerful tool for health in the hands of ordinary patients. It would be a fair summary to say that for many maladies there are many potential benefits and many uncertainties, and that the strongest conclusion is that more research is essential to identify, enhance, and exploit these benefits, and to reduce those uncertainties (Beratarrechea et al. 2014; Joe and Demiris 2013; Or and Tao 2014; Petersen and DeMuro 2015; cf. World Health Organization 2011).

Suppose it is determined that mobile tools and the Internet are improving health care. Is that improvement at an acceptable cost? We should explore this question in some detail. At ground, e-, m-, and tele-health have evolved quickly not because a careful evaluation or needs assessment concluded, for instance, "Use more telephones to help people look up symptoms on the Web." All the electronic ecosystems in communications, business, and health expanded rapidly because they provided something people wanted and were willing to pay for. Ubiquitous connectivity has both changed civilization and challenged it in vastly many ways. As is usually the case, a technology advanced rapidly – in the case of informa-tion technology, with unprecedented rapidity – and we later came to wonder if, or how, it should be governed, and by whom. But this means that the new technology infiltrates and alters existing processes and ways of doing business without clear warrant that it will be for the better. Maybe, that is, we should have improved what we started with.[3] If people have limited access to health care, then perhaps the best course is to improve access to health care, not adopt a new technology of cameras and sensors and hope that it will improve things. Indeed, it might indeed improve some things, but at the price of losing or diminishing something we had good antecedent reason to value. The clinician–patient relationship is a good example of this. As we saw in Chapter 2, the price of a flawless diagnostic Professor Robodoc might be too dear if it comes at the expense of that relationship.

The case of telehealth, or "remote-presence health care," including telemedicine, serves as an exemplar. It was perhaps inevitable that the availability of high-speed digital tools would inspire caregivers for prisoners, people in rural areas, soldiers, and even astronauts to desire and then develop tools to try to care for people at a distance (Clark et al. 2010).[4] The first telehealth interventions were provided before a single randomized trial or case-control study. They just made a kind of sense in the context: It is difficult, impossible, or inconvenient to be there, so surely the next best thing would be to use television and the Internet. The most visually oriented practices (dermatology,[5] pathology, psychiatry,[6] and radiology) were pioneers. Great progress has apparently ensued, although it has been challenged, as in much biomedical research, by important debates about the quality of efforts to study outcomes and effectiveness (Law and Wason 2014). The denouement is that we have somehow managed to bootstrap the use and acceptance of a new technology without the usual kind of evidence base on which we otherwise tend to insist. It might, that is, have been best for society to have given prisoners or residents of rural areas traditional standard-of-care health interventions. That we were unwilling to do this means that aspects of telehealth, however good it is, sometimes sidestep the varieties of moral urgency that customarily inspire progressive change.

The telehealth literature emphasizes ethical issues related to confidentiality and legal issues of reimbursement, cross-border practice, and credentialing. The World Medical Association, however, seems to draw a distinction between telehealth by necessity and telehealth by convenience: "The patient-physician relationship should be based on a personal encounter and sufficient knowledge of the patient's personal history. Telemedicine should be employed primarily in situations in which a physician cannot be physically present within a safe and acceptable time period."[7] This appeal to the clinician–patient relationship is reaffirmed as a kind of moral safe harbor in the face of challenges by incipient technologies.

Unfortunately, in the case of much mobile health, there was no such relationship in the first place. The use of mobile health technologies, then, emerges as a kind of surrender to our inability to improve things otherwise. Its use becomes an instance of telehealth by necessity, born of our failure to do better. This is a very weak kind of "necessity." It is an opportunity to prevent the perfect from being the enemy of the good. If at the end of the day, or century, we find that this good was not good enough, then it will be too late: We will wish society had done a better job providing humans to take care of sick people in the first place.

Digital and other divides

If mobile technologies impede or prevent improvement of health care or its systems, we should perhaps be relieved if people in low socioeconomic groups have less access to them. If, however, there is evidence that these technologies have positive effects, then we will have created or worsened yet another class-based disparity. There is, in any event, at least some evidence in support of the utility of mobile health technologies in resource-limited regions, including some in high-income countries (recall the discussion of electronic health record use in low- and middle-income countries from Chapter 1). Moreover, it has been wisely suggested, our ordinary ideas of what should count as "access" to care must themselves evolve: "As the paradigm of healthcare delivery evolves towards greater reliance on non-encounter-based digital communications between patients and their care teams, it is critical that our theoretical conceptualization of access undergoes a concurrent paradigm shift to make it more relevant for the digital age" (Fortney et al. 2011, S639). Current definitions of access are exclusively of face-to-face encounters, leading to a proposed new definition: "Access to care represents the potential ease of having virtual or face-to-face interactions with a broad array of healthcare providers including clinicians, caregivers, peers, and computer applications" (ibid.). But that is about access to care. Access to the Internet is another matter. Digital divides are very difficult to assess across populations, and, moreover, the availability of mobile digital technology has surpassed that of desktop bandwidth and function established in high-resource regions. Put differently, even people in low-income and low-resource regions have mobile phones, and these are potentially rich sources of access to health information and advice. While independent, that is, nonindustry, surveys of mobile device access are difficult to acquire, it is in bounds to consider, first, that the number of mobile phones was expected to exceed the world's population in 2014[8] and, moreover, that 90% of people in the world at least 6 years old will have a mobile phone, and there will be 6.1 billion smartphone subscriptions, by the year 2020 (up from 2.7 billion in 2014).[9]

Even commitments to transparency, veracity, and accountability might be inadequate to this task. That is, it might be that even if a corporation or an industry commits to these value standards, users will still not receive what they need for health maintenance or improved health.

No matter the users' socioeconomic status, according to one team, there is "little or no quality control or regulation ... to ensure health apps are user-friendly, accurate in content, evidence-based, or efficacious" (Boudreaux et al. 2014, 364). To our three emphasized values, we might consider adding a fourth: quality. Of concern for decades, the Web-based information that really matters remains of variable quality (e.g., Scullard et al. 2010). Seeking to address this, the team offers the following context: There are:

> four categories of virtual healthcare utilization that should be considered in addition to traditional encounters: (1) synchronous digital patient-to-provider encounters, (2) asynchronous digital patient-to-provider communications, (3) digital peer-to-peer communications, and (4) synchronous digital interactions between patients and computer health applications. Digital communication modalities currently include cell phones, smartphones, interactive voice response, text messages, e-mails, interactive video, web-cams, personal monitoring devices, kiosks, personal health records, web-based portals, social networking sites, secure chat rooms, and on-line forums. These e-health technologies enable synchronous and asynchronous digital communications between patients and their formal providers, informal caregivers, peers, and computer applications and allow face-to-face patient-to-provider encounters to focus on medical procedures requiring physical proximity and tactile contact. (ibid.)

Boudreaux and colleagues then offer seven approaches or strategies for review and assessment. These strategies parallel and embrace the demand for system evaluation laid out in Chapter 2:

> (1) Review the scientific literature, (2) Search app clearinghouse Web sites, (3) Search app stores, (4) Review app descriptions, user ratings, and reviews, (5) Conduct a social media query in professional and, if available, patient networks, (6) Pilot the apps, and (7) Elicit feedback from patients. (ibid.)

Add to this the idea that "virtual advisors" who delivered "culturally and linguistically adapted" health promotion advice might improve uptake and outcomes and help address, if not manage, some disparities (King et al. 2013).

This is an opportunity for sustained innovation, focused research, and creative application. The translational research movement would do well to include mobile health and consumer health informatics in its ambit. From the global Web to a child's cellphone, the matrix of health information and advice has changed the way rich and poor try to make sense of illness and disability. Although health information technology raises profound ethical issues for all populations, these issues are often lensed by poverty, class, and deprivation. It would be a tragic mistake if we were to be so enthralled by our digital gadgets that we forgot Simon's lesson, that "a wealth of information creates a poverty of attention" – and somehow came to believe we had done our duty without enhancing nutrition, primary care, and bona fide health literacy or, in other populations, ensuring access to clean water, vaccinations, and basic education.

Generic top-level domains

If so much of our attention is drawn to the role of the Internet and World Wide Web as sources or failures of transparency, veracity, accountability, and quality, it would be well to review one of the most interesting and contentious issues that has evolved regarding its governance and the role of health on the net.

Before 1998, there were eight "generic top-level domain names," or gTLDs, the last part of the uniform resource locator, or URL, that constitutes an address on the World Wide Web: .com, .edu, .gov, .int, .mil, .net, .org, and .arpa. The Advanced Research Projects Agency (ARPA) was a US Defense Department unit where computer scientists' work on signal processing led to the creation of ARPANET for research and academic use; it evolved into the Internet. (It is now DARPA, for Defense Advanced Research Projects Agency.) A single ARPA computer scientist, Jon Postel, had the task of cataloging what are known as "Internet Protocol" (IP) numbers for individual and groups of computers; he also had a role in creating the language- (i.e., not number) based system of domain names. The process seemed and sounded so modest and ad hoc that it was named the Internet Assigned Numbers Authority (Zittrain 2014).[10] This organization, in turn, evolved into the Internet Corporation for Assigned Names and Numbers (ICANN), founded in 1998.

In 2000, ICANN rejected the World Health Organization[11] and consumer groups' application for a "dedicated and safe space for health information" on the Internet – ".health" (Mackey et al. 2013, 1404; cf. Illman 2000). An expansion of top-level domain names begun in 2012 engendered a tense debate over e-health governance. Top-level domain names are auctioned, with brokers bidding against each other, generally on behalf of clients; the application fee alone is $185,000. An extraordinary dispute was over the question whether a for-profit company with no background in health should own ".health" (dot-health). Objections emphasized these concerns: There was no active participation in the auction by public health stakeholders, likely because the price is too high for such; the major players were entrepreneurs from high-income countries with exclusively commercial interests; and there are no provisions required for consumer protection (Mackey et al. 2014). The overarching concern, however, was this: .health (and perhaps .santé, .salud, .saúde, etc.) carries special meaning, unique importance, and greater responsibility. It would be very unfortunate, indeed, it was argued, if a tobacco cartel, liquor firm, or laetrile vendor were to own it.

Although there is little to mull over .cricket, .baseball, .charity, or .flowers, say, then surely, it was argued, judgment could be applied when the stakes were higher.[12] A variety of public health and professional organizations contended unsuccessfully that, at the least, there should be a moratorium on the sale of .health. Most disputes over top-level domain assignment were based on competing stakeholders (e.g., .radio, .green, .church), whereas the contention here was between stakeholders and nonstakeholders. Why does that matter? According to the World Health Organization:

A trusted environment for the health Internet is essential and fully achievable. It is critical to health security, health and medical education, the protection of privacy and the promotion of public health on a societal scale. Health is a highly-regulated sector in most countries. However, the global nature of the Internet makes national laws difficult to enforce. Therefore, it is imperative that the management and operation of health-related generic top-level domains (gTLDs), including .health, be consistent with public health objectives in order to serve the public, civil society, governments and industry on a global scale.

(World Health Organization 2014)

The worst that could happen is that a highest bidder might find good financial reasons to forgo Geneva's demands that several criteria be met, including governance and management, transparency, privacy and security, and global services: "Establishing much-needed governing principles for the .health gTLD is the key to ensuring the Internet can play its proper role in supporting global public health" (ibid.). The World Health Organization also suggested that a .health domain could be a valuable and trusted medium for exchanging "sensitive health information" during emergencies.

One way to view the sale of top-level domain names is as a kind of privatization of that which is essentially and unalterably public. Unlike radio frequencies, for instance, there is no limit on the number of available channels. Contrarily, the power of a term or phrase or word considerably narrows the width of available channels. Indeed, ICANN does have criteria for vetting applications and it takes into account whether, in fact, someone has any credibility in speaking for, or claiming to be able to represent, a group. This many-edged knife is of a brand unlikely to produce a cut that will satisfy everyone. What is not unreasonable, given that the stakes are plausibly of great importance to public health, is that when the scope is broad enough, important enough, and risky enough, there is a very powerful case to be made to prefer organizations with long international track records in the salient domain. There is little chance that will happen to be the highest bidder.

Social networking

For all the well-motivated (but asynchronous) wringing of hands, biting of nails, and beating of breasts over privacy and data protection, it is a never-ending source of wonder how freely some people share their personal, even intimate, information. From the earliest e-mail and bulletin board systems and chat rooms, to microblogs, social networking sites, and wikis, the lure and allure of life online is, for many, a temptation they are unable to resist. It might be possible to infer that otherwise keen attention to privacy is demoted in exchange for access to new technologies and the benefits they are believed to deliver. But first:

Social media are Web-based tools that are used for computer-mediated communication. In health care, they have been used to maintain or improve peer-to-peer and clinician-to-patient communication, promote institutional branding, and improve the speed of interaction between and across different health care stakeholders. Examples of social media applications in health include (but are not limited to) access to educational resources by clinicians and patients, generation of content rich reference resources (eg, Wikipedia), evaluation and reporting of real-time flu trends, catalyzing outreach during (public) health campaigns, and recruitment of patients to online studies and in clinical trials.

A number of indicators suggest that the evidence for using social media in the health care context is growing; for example, the number of articles indexed on PubMed has nearly doubled each year for the last 4 years, social media policies are being adopted and tested in various health care settings, journals are discussing how social media facilitate knowledge-sharing and collaboration, and theories on the social changes resulting from their adoption are being developed. However, despite these useful insights, our collective understanding of how social media can be used in medical and health care remains fragmented.

(Grajales et al. 2014; cf. Farmer et al. 2009; Winkelstein 2013)

Social media, that is, have become embedded in our strategies for coping with illness. We – some of us, anyway – seek information, advice, and comfort; others share, publish, and disclose, perhaps to therapeutic advantage. The issues that confront us are in some respects of a piece with ancient challenges, and "in many ways similar to issues that physicians and medical institutions have dealt with for generations. Physicians, after all, are members of real-life communities and might be observed in public behaving in ways that are discordant with their professional personas" (Jain 2009, 650). Physicians, nurses, and psychologists have friends outside their practices, and many are challenged by boundary issues such as those that arise when one seeks professional advice. With family members and actual friends, that is almost always a bad idea (Eastwood 2009). According to the American College of Physicians, "Physicians should usually not enter into the dual relationship of physician-family member or physician-friend for a variety of reasons. The patient may be at risk of receiving inferior care from the physician. Problems may include effects on clinical objectivity, inadequate history-taking or physical examination, over-testing, inappropriate prescribing, incomplete counseling on sensitive issues, or failure to keep appropriate medical records" (Snyder 2012).

Indeed, that is for actual *friends*. As has become commonplace to note, the meaning of "friend" has devolved such that, for many of us, any passerby who clicks on the appropriate link can be termed a "friend." If treating a real friend is a mistake, surely "friending" a patient, or allowing oneself to be "friended" – this awful verb notwithstanding – is a worse mistake. According to the American College of Physicians: "Professional distance and privacy are appropriate for both physician and patient. Physicians should not 'friend' or contact patients through personal social media. Physicians should familiarize themselves with the privacy settings and terms of agreements for social media platforms to which they subscribe, and they should maintain strict privacy settings on personal accounts. Professional profiles should be constructed with an explicit purpose (such as networking and community outreach)" (Farnan et al. 2013, 624). This world is changing rapidly, and the number of clinicians with social media accounts is likewise changing rapidly. While as many as 96% of health science students had Facebook accounts at one point, fewer than half of all professional clinicians did (von Muhlen and Ohno-Machado 2012).

This is a good place to emphasize that these are interesting challenges, perhaps problems, certainly sources of controversy – but they are not "dilemmas," in the overused and often misplaced locution (a "dilemma," recall, being an intractable conflict, and, in ethics, a situation such that no matter what one does, one does something wrong). The *reasons* why a nurse or physician should not friend a patient include that it is not an established medium for professional communication, it risks misunderstandings, it enjoys no research basis for utility in clinical practice, and, unlike personal health records (as we saw in Chapter 1), it includes no ground rules or provisions to protect confidentiality or reassure patients (Househ et al. 2014) and no prior education to ensure best practice. These are good reasons, and that is sound guidance.

How are social media different than e-mail or text messaging? This is not clear. While electronic mail is perhaps more like a telephone call or even a letter, its use is not established and there are no norms to guide its use. In other words, we do not know enough (Atherton et al. 2012). This means that any use of e-mail between patient and clinician must be carefully circumscribed and both parties must agree to its scope and applicability. An e-mail might prevent the need for an office visit, suggesting possible cost-savings, but it can also seem to require a detailed and carefully written response, which a clinician is likely to disdain. The fact that e-mail is asynchronous is a drawback and source of risk. The concept of "progressive caution," advanced in Chapter 1, should provide guidance here. Move slowly, learn more, and avoid unnecessary risk.[13]

It is perhaps the second item just noted that is of the greatest importance. In the same way fledgling nurses and physicians are trained – or should be trained – to communicate with patients and to enter notes in charts, we must identify best practices and develop curricula so that the use of social media becomes part of professional clinicians' skill set (Brown et al. 2014). Our inclination to bootstrap new technology merely because we fancy it will work every so often, but to make a habit of this is to play fast and loose with patient safety, public health, and professional stances acquired over a very long time.

This is emphatically not to say that we must turn away from potentially innovative technologies. If social media can support research (see Chapter 8), improve organ donation rates (Sadler and Sadler 2012), contribute to community education and consultation (Galbraith 2014), and improve behavior change (Laranjo et al. 2014), then we will have used health information technology for the better. This, of course, has been the goal all along.

Sousveillance, medical homes, and robots

The physical presence of another human is not necessary for at least some measure of health care. We've seen that with enough cameras and sensors, it is possible to provide "remote presence" or "telehealth care" in which a clinician at a distance can interview, look at, advise, and otherwise provide a first approximation of an assessment; some might even call it an "examination." Furthermore, a living human, if monitored, generates a great deal of data, and we now have the ability to acquire and analyze it, all of it. To be sure, people now can monitor themselves to improve or maintain fitness, and as long as applications that track miles walked, blood pressure, or pulse rate do not mislead someone who needs medical attention, this is probably a virtue. But we should consider a world of pervasive or ubiquitous data collection and monitoring, and a world in which robots, perhaps androids or those that appear as human, and digital companions interact with humans to provide assistance, some of it emotional. In both cases, the patient could be or is disconnected from any traditional "point of care" and, indeed, in principle, from any human.

Sousveillance, quantified selves, and medical homes

Begin with what has come to be called the "quantified self," a movement to celebrate the large-scale collection and analysis of personal data about health and other aspects of individuals for their well-being and that of populations (Swan 2009, 2012a, 2012b). Add a complement of wearable and other sensors. Include whole genome sequencing. If fully realized for enough people, this could constitute the largest source of big health data, ever. Then provide health coaches to guide the people who were the source of the data, better to make the most of it in support of their wellness. There is, of course, a project to attempt this, that is, to focus on "optimizing wellness through longitudinal data collection, integration and mining of individual data clouds, enabling development of predictive models of wellness and disease that will reveal actionable possibilities," where this would be accomplished by:

> gathering data in four main areas: (1) whole genome sequencing; (2) clinical and functional laboratory testing (every three months); (3) gut microbiome (every three months); and (4) quantified self and traits (physical activity, sleep, weight, blood pressure, personality and lifestyle factors, and so on). Once the results are returned, health coaches work with participants on a monthly basis to identify priority areas for lifestyle change or make referrals to physicians if medical follow-up is warranted. In addition to the data for which we are coaching, we are measuring a variety of proteomic and metabolomics markers as part of a scientific discovery effort. (Hood et al. 2015)

This is both exciting and alarming. It is exciting because it suggests a smart way to identify, collect, and parse data in the service of better health. What could be better? It is alarming because such data suction constitutes progress toward a fantastic world of ubiquitous surveillance and what has been called "pervasive information and communication technologies." Thus, "PICT is variously termed ubiquitous computing (or ubicomp), pervasive computing, everywhere, and ambient intelligence (AmI). The four adjectives – 'ubiquitous,' 'pervasive,' 'every(where),' and 'ambient' – highlight the expected omnipresence of these devices, being embedded in and just about everything found just about anywhere" (Pimple 2014, 2).[14] Imagine wearing clothes with physiologic sensors and radio frequency identification chips (Glasser et al. 2007), shoes with balance – or off-balance – detectors, in a room with motion detectors and, for that matter, cameras with image-analysis software, linked to a smartphone and to an electronic health record with genomic data – and all of it stored in a cloud and being monitored and analyzed by a person or a machine somewhere else. Do not stop at wearable devices: Progress in development of "bioelectronics medicines" or "electroceuticals" entails progress in being able to monitor internal physiologic and other functions and states (Rogers 2015). Indeed, imagine being 85 years old and having it all paid for as a social benefit on which you insisted. The gap between the excitement of having your life saved if you fell and the disquiet of being so comprehensively observed that it just isn't worth it should be mapped and bridged with thoughtful and nuanced rules and policies. This approach is especially apt for products with great potential and great uncertainty about safety, a Web-connected and implanted drug delivery system, for instance (Farra et al. 2012). Even without such safeguards, however, some of us will be delighted to sign on the dotted line.

This tension parallels the one we face in larger civil society in trying to balance the benefits of corporate or governmental monitoring with the moral and sometimes political offensiveness of the intrusion needed to achieve the benefit. Police states have less crime.

"Sousveillance" is, generally, the *self*-monitoring or recording of a behavior, physiological state, or environment. (*Surveillance* is, generally, monitoring by someone else.) Data thus acquired can be transmitted and analyzed. It should be uncontroversial to affirm that an extraordinarily good justification is needed to require someone to conduct sousveillance, that is, monitor herself digitally and share the results. Now consider a severely demented patient being cared for under the principle of "least restrictive" oversight. Would a wearable camera, which the person does not understand and might not be aware of, be an acceptable form of sousveillance if the intent of its use is to protect the person from others who might be a source of harm, or from various forms of self-neglect or injury? (Cf. Freshwater et al. 2013) What about an implanted monitoring device?

Although it is customary to include human intentions as part of comprehensive ethical analyses, even good intentions might be inadequate to prepare or guide us. Indeed, this is the challenge of many new technologies: We should assume that all those who are keen to adopt the new technologies intend to do good. It is when we fail to apply additional moral filters that we risk ethical trouble. So it is well to be concerned about the kind and magnitude of the trade-offs being contemplated:

> Many [pervasive information and communication] technologies take action only when initiated by a human, or as a response to strictly defined circumstances more-or-less after the fashion of a smoke detector. Others, however, take action based on their own analysis of complex, quickly changing, or multiple streams of data, as in high-frequency trading ... In some cases these systems raise issues beyond privacy and deception to serious physical, social, and economic harms. [Artificial intelligence] systems are increasingly making life-and-death and/or multi-million dollar decisions without direct human intervention or adequate supervision.
> (Pimple 2014, 3)

There are several ways to begin to approach this challenge. The first is to curb our enthusiasm about the likely utility of any of this. Actual benefit will require years of research and evaluation to achieve. Second, we just earlier mulled a "data collection, integration and mining of individual data clouds" project that included health coaches, that is, which included human intervention in a key role. It is likely that for some sousveillance tools we also must titrate our expectations so that wearable devices enable or foster changes in health behavior, for instance – but are alone unable to impel or drive that change (Patel et al. 2015). Third, it is overoptimistic to suppose that a set of (ethics) rules will be adequate to ensure the benefits of a technology while preventing abuses. What is needed also is a system of governance informed by those rules. (We will take up the uses of "trusted governance" in Chapter 8.)

Perhaps the best example of this is in the development of "medical homes" or dwellings specially equipped to foster health, usually either for elders or people with chronic disease. The evidence so far is suggestive, even encouraging, of a medical home resource as long as it is operated under some form of credible oversight (Rosenthal 2008) and, especially, as regards communication with caregivers, as the locus for more research (Walsh et al. 2013). From adults with chronic conditions and frail elders to adolescent substance abusers and children with special needs, the idea of digital medical homes is both tempting and under-supported (Jackson et al. 2013).

Robots and digital companions

There are other ways of being remote, disconnected, or at a distance. Consider the following argument:

> Humans have duties to care for each other, especially loved ones.
> Those duties ought generally not be delegated to proxies.
> Therefore, to delegate a caregiving duty to a proxy is generally a shirking of a duty to loved ones.

It is a simple albeit vague syllogism, but it captures a common, uncontroversial intuition, namely that the act of caring for someone else is the fulfillment of a human duty or obligation. At its weakest, the obligation entails the following:

- Parents have duties to care for their children.
- Children have duties to care for their parents.
- Family members have duties to care for each other.

Stronger versions might entail these requirements:

- Neighbors have duties to care for each other.
- Citizens have duties to care for each other.
- Humans have duties to care for each other.

Now, by "care for" we must mean – well, what exactly? To feed? Shelter? Comfort? Clean? The question is murkier when we consider the complexity in mapping duties to needs. Must a child always feed and clean a parent in need? A spouse? If not always, when? And under what circumstances? What was an uncontroversial intuition a moment ago is now perhaps the source of some discomfort: If we say a child must feed a parent whose disability prevents Dad from lifting a spoon, we surely cannot fault the son or daughter from arranging for a trusted agent – a staffer in a skilled nursing facility, for instance, or a home health aide – to feed the parent. To say, as we did above, that "Children have duties to care for their parents" certainly cannot require that all children must learn to tend to Mom's intimate personal hygiene needs. And some people do not have children, spouses, or other such potential caregivers.

What we want to say in such cases is that contemporary civil society has some responsibility to help ordinary people meet their duties to others. We could debate the extent and scope of such services. But those whose politico-economic compasses always turn against public support for personal needs – those who disdain publicly supported health care, childcare, and eldercare – libertarians, survivalists, and other anti-social-service zealots whom we visited in Chapter 6 now have the assignment of providing a moral defense of such indignity and neglect as follows from their policies.

What about robots? Computer-assisted and human-controlled robotic tools have become a feature of many medical centers, apparently to good or at least acceptable effect (Kumar and Asaf 2015). Consisting in arrays of precision instruments with a number of "arms" with devices to cut, cauterize, and photograph, these devices are operated by surgeons. The machines cancel hand trembling and can be set to change the scale of the procedure; that is, what takes place in a patient in millimeters can be scaled up on a display to several centimeters or larger, in principle, improving laparoscopic procedures. Data about outcomes (prostatectomies, hysterectomies, and mitral valve repair are common uses) should guide ethical analysis, although it is reasonable to inquire whether any improvement in outcomes is equal to any increase in health care costs. These devices cost some $2 million each, with high maintenance expenses.

Now, what about robotic caregivers?

The possibility of being cared for exclusively by robots is no longer science fiction. There has been a dramatic increase in the number of companies producing robots for the care or companionship, or both, of the elderly and children. A number of robot manufacturers in South Korea and Japan are racing to fulfill the dream of affordable robot "nannies." These have video game playing, quizzes, speech recognition, face recognition, and limited conversation to capture the preschool child's interest and attention. Their mobility and semi-autonomous functions, combined with facilities for visual and auditory monitoring by the carer, are designed to keep the child from harm. These are very tempting for busy, professional parents. Most of the robots are prohibitively expensive at present, but prices are falling and some cheap versions are already becoming available. (Sharkey and Sharkey 2012, 267)

One response to this development is to mourn the evolution of societies in which parents are too busy to care for their children and society itself is unable or unwilling to help; another is to invoke the distinction between tools of necessity and those of convenience, and insist on the former as a justification for any nontrivial role of robots in human health care. Surely we would salute a Robodoc that saved a wounded soldier or dying astronaut. We could also sigh and surrender to another suite of economically driven gadgets on which we come to depend after not really needing them in the first place.[15]

Suppose, however, that an intelligent robot – imagine a humanoid device, or android – were able to interact with an autistic child, using games, songs, and language, to good effect (cf. Mushiaki 2013)? Or a "carebot" that improved an elder's mobility or eating (Cornet 2013). What if, that is, the robot could exceed human abilities? Some scholars draw a distinction among "shallow," "good," and "deep" care, such that shallow care is routine, good care "respects human dignity," and deep care requires reciprocity of feelings between care recipient and caregiver (Coeckelbergh 2010, 185). The notion that a computational entity might have feelings need not detain us. What we want is guidance for development and use of those entities in health care. Jason Borenstein and Yvette Pearson, via Coeckelbergh, suggest that if a robot can be of physical and/or emotional use or assistance, then what is now generally called "human-robot interaction" (e.g., Datteri 2013) might or will improve to the point that, "Assuming that it is not inherently undignified to be cared for by a robot, the absence of 'deep' care does not entail the absence of 'good' care" (Borenstein and Pearson 2012, 255).[16] In the event it is true that the deep should not be the enemy of the good, we again acquire the assignment to evaluate and study these new technologies with the same ardor as we buy them.

What are called "socially intelligent robots" or "cognitive robot companions" have elicited an interest in their "social behavior" and even rules to guide it (Dautenhahn 2007). (We anticipated this in Chapter 6 (note 4) with a citation of Isaac Asimov's three "Laws of Robotics.") As artificial intelligence has advanced, we face, or will soon face, human-appearing machines that process and produce speech and express what seem to be emotions and other mental states. A robot might express empathy. Is this an acceptable substitute for a human, and does it matter if that human is alone in the world, without family, unbefriended? Indeed, is this an ethical issue or an aesthetic one? There is something uncanny, outré, or even creepy about a human-like but nonliving thing seeming to communicate, console, or help a human.[17] But that is perhaps only when first learning about them:[18]

When robots make eye contact, recognize faces, mirror human gestures, they push our Darwinian buttons, exhibiting the kinds of behavior people associate with sentience, intentions, and emotions. Once people see robots as creatures, people feel a desire to nurture them. With this feeling comes the fantasy of reciprocation: as we begin to care for robots, we want them to care about us. In our nascent robotics culture, nurturance turns out to be a "killer app". Eleven-year-old Fara reacts to a play session with Cog, a humanoid robot at MIT that can meet her eyes, follow her position and imitate her movements, by saying that she could never get tired of the robot because "it's not like a toy because you can't teach a toy; it's like something that's part of you, you know, something you love, kind of like another person, like a baby." (Turkle 2010, 3–4)

Yorick Wilks, a leader in natural language processing and machine translation, writes of "machine conversationalists" as heirs to "entertaining" 1960s efforts such as Joseph Weizenbaum's ELIZA program to simulate a psychotherapist: A working digital companion "would learn its person's likes and dislikes, carry out Web-related tasks accordingly, and prompt reminiscences about the person's photo collection so as to build up his or her life story through conversation"(Wilks 2007, 928). He makes clear that a barrier to previous natural language-processing analyses has been a lack of easily acquirable examples of human speech and communication, and that the World Wide Web constitutes an ultravast repository of examples.

Beyond assistance in living, a "mechanical assisted intimacy device" might comfort the dying. A prototype, conceived of as an art installation, has an actuator connected to a cloth pad that strokes a simulated hospice patient's arm. The device includes a voice recording:

> Hello Susie, I am the Last Moment Robot. I am here to help you and guide you through your last moment on earth. I am sorry that your family and friends can't be with you right now, but don't be afraid. I am here to comfort you. You are not alone, you are with me. Your family and friends love you very much, they will remember you after you are gone. Time of death 11:56.[19]

Perhaps elders, children, and the dying will value this attention. Perhaps someone who is lonely or sick will conclude that a digital companion is better than nothing. Perhaps we will find that digital companions, like pets, are good for improving emotional states and even physical well-being (Urbanski and Lazenby 2012). If we are to consider such "digital companion therapy" seriously, we will need to resolve several issues, many of which are familiar but which have a flavor completely different from their antecedents.

Consent: What information should be shared with someone to be outfitted with a digital companion or, for that matter, to be placed in a digital home? Will the patient (or a surrogate or proxy) be able to refuse?

Confidentiality: If one confides in an intelligent machine companion, does it have duties to protect that information? What if the patient confides something such that if it were shared with a human would trigger a clinical response or warning, perhaps to someone else?

Trust and communication: The foundations of most successful clinical relationships, including trust and communication, cannot yet be replicated in a machine. That is, a "relationship" generally requires reciprocity. Is it deceptive to induce the belief that one has a relationship with a robot, digital companion, or machine conversationalist?

It has been suggested that some cultures, those, for instance, which embrace various forms of animism, will adopt robotic tools more readily than others (Mushiaki 2013). Good explanations are not necessarily good warrants or justifications, however. Cultures that are racist, sexist, or ageist, for instance, are not merely local variations in the moral tapestry – they are misguided and mistaken. It is a meta-empirical question whether the growth of robots and digital companions can be accompanied by insightful ethics, adequate governance, and a commitment to self-correcting research. If we have agreed on anything so far, it is this: The ethical care of humans is often a matter of finding warrant to change a standard. Such warrant is often and itself acquired (or not) through more research. The decoupling of patient and clinician, either because of distance or absence, is a challenge requiring no less formal inquiry than any other putatively beneficial alteration in the way we live, ail, and die.

Notes

1. Nevertheless, try this: Select any browser and enter a string of symptoms; include some attributable to a pet. Whether one actually learns anything, or receives practical guidance, is precisely among the issues to be mooted.

2. According to McDaid and Park (2011, 12), the Chinese Web site www.cnkang.com is "Fully accessible using a mobile phone, it provides information on healthy diet, disease-related knowledge and self-diagnosis tools about, for example, how to diagnose diabetes. It also includes interactive options allowing individuals to join virtual communities or consult medical experts online." As to reliability, it should perhaps be noted that a section on men's health is for some reason illustrated with a photo of a supine young male. Standing next to him is a woman who has placed one foot, in a red boot with a very long heel, on his abdomen; the Chinese caption apparently reads "male prepuce risk."

3. Indeed, we now have criteria for evaluating and choosing mobile apps: "(1) Review the scientific literature, (2) Search app clearinghouse Web sites, (3) Search app stores, (4) Review app descriptions, user ratings, and reviews, (5) Conduct a social media query within professional and, if available, patient networks, (6) Pilot the apps, and (7) Elicit feedback from patients" (Boudreaux et al. 2014, 364).

4. According to Clark et al. (2010, 262):

    Applications of telemedicine were first seen as early as 1877 with the use of the telephone. At this time, twenty-one doctors practicing medicine in nearby areas developed a communication system with a local drugstore via telephone lines. Later, in 1927, the first live video consult between a patient and a physician occurred, known as the "radio doctor". In the 1950s in the form of two-way television group therapy, diagnoses were given via videotaped recordings and satellite communication for rural health care in Alaska [notes omitted].

5. There has been such progress in teledermatology that it now seems to make sense to address access to *it* in addition to traditional access to a physician (Shannon and Buker 2010).

6. Behavioral health presents special problems, not addressed in detail here. At ground, the question for psychologists and psychiatrists is whether an online encounter ("e-therapy") is an adequate facsimile of face-to-face interactions. Although it is difficult to see how a sufficient and appropriate therapeutic relationship can be built with a patient or client one has never met in person, this is an empirical question. See Manhal-Baugus (2001) for a discussion.

7. World Medical Association, www.wma.net/en/30publications/10policies/t3/. It is probably uncontroversial to suggest that telehealth resources should be used as much as possible to contribute to care of critical-care patients with, say, Ebola. The virtue in such a case would be that, if an adequate level of care can be provided, there accrues the additional benefit of reducing risk to caregivers.

8. "World to have more cell phone accounts than people by 2014," *siliconindia Magazines*, 2 January 2013, available at www.siliconindia.com/magazine_articles/World_to_have_more_cell_phone_accounts_than_people_by_2014-DASD767476836.html.

9. "Ericsson: 90% of world's population will have a mobile phone by 2020," FierceWirelessEurope, 19 November 2014, available at www.fiercewireless.com/europe/story/ericsson-90-cent-worlds-population-will-have-mobile-phone-2020/2014-11-19.

10. See Postel (1994), where he lays out what may be taken to be a draft of the architecture for the future Internet. Correct and wise about so much, he was delightfully wrong in one prediction:

    In the Domain Name System (DNS) naming of computers there is a hierarchy of names. The root of system is unnamed. There are a set of what are called "top-level domain names" (TLDs). These are the generic TLDs (EDU, COM, NET, ORG, GOV, MIL, and INT), and the two letter country codes from ISO-3166. It is extremely unlikely that any other TLDs will be created.

11. The author of this volume is the director of a WHO Collaborating Centre for Ethics and Global Health Policy and he traveled at WHO expense to a meeting to discuss the dot-health issue in Geneva in December 2013. He received and receives no personal compensation for either effort.

12. On the other hand, the Internet Corporation for Assigned Names and Numbers approved ".sucks" (whose buyer proclaimed its "intention from the very beginning to operate [the domain] with integrity [and] respect for the security and stability of the internet ...") and ".wtf" ("as an expression of disbelief, anger, or astonishment ... a flexible and creative alternative to the TLD norm").

13. One disconcerting risk is that any extended use of social media for clinical purposes might itself contribute to a behavioral malady – in our case, what has been termed "Facebook addiction" (Ryan et al. 2014).

14. Professor Pimple's collection is a valuable introduction to challenges posed by these pervasive technologies. He summarizes elsewhere three of PICT's distinguishing characteristics:

    - It is, or could be, anywhere and everywhere – buildings, billboards, floors, restrooms, purses, pockets, coffee makers, pacemakers, eyeglasses, and the kitchen sink.
    - It detects, collects, organizes, acts upon, and transmits information, often wirelessly on the Internet.
    - Its presence and operation [are] often undetected by casual users, whether hidden physically (e.g., computer chips embedded in automobiles) or functionally. Functional invisibility occurs when a function or use of the technology is not announced (e.g., tracking online behavior), announced in a cryptic fashion (as in most terms of use), or becomes ambient through a process of familiarization, such as when smartphones become as ordinary as wallets and Facebook becomes a way of life. (available at http://ethicalpait.blogspot.com/2014/03/what-is-pervasive-ict.html)

15. See Anderson and Anderson (2011) and Lin et al. (2012) for thoughtful collections of analyses of "robot ethics" and related issues.

16. The role and status of "dignity" is complex. It has been suggested that human life without some indignity is unavoidable, that it is a "squishy, subjective notion, hardly up to the heavyweight moral demands assigned to it," and that its invocation is as often a political ploy as a commitment to something of value (Pinker 2008). There is, for instance, precious little "dignity" in many ordinary clinical encounters and hospital stays, even in an environment of committed, professional, and respectful caregivers. We often interpret unavoidable affronts to modesty or pride as indignities, but surely that can contain little moral weight.

17. Perhaps well-trained zombies might be of use; see Greene and Mo (2006) for assessments of philosophical issues and the undead. Zombies are universally portrayed as behaving badly, despite their apparent lack of any ability to have any intentions other than to eat the hero. But surely there could be nice and even nurturing zombies. Indeed, "Zombie Nanny" would make a splendid title. (Having just made that up, I find that a search in a common browser returns some 2,000 instances of it. Such is the World Wide Web, not to mention delusions of unique cleverness.)

18. Or perhaps there is something fundamentally misguided about this entire enterprise. The inventor and entrepreneur Elon Musk, who has invested in artificial intelligence, has expressed concern about the unregulated technology: "With artificial intelligence we are summoning the demon. In all those stories where there's the guy with the pentagram and the holy water, it's like – yeah, he's sure he can control the demon. Doesn't work out" (Gibbs 2014).

19. The "Last Moment Robot" is the creation of Dan Chen, whose Rhode Island School of Design master of fine art thesis, "File > Save As > Intimacy: What Is Intimacy without Humanity?" challenges views about the connection between the two. From the Web site: "As sculptural studies and experience designs, these devices reveal how [robot intimacy technology] might work for us; as transitional objects providing an emotional placebo effect, instead of emotional life support." See www.pixedge.com/lastmoment.
    We need not stop at death. Robot-mediated sex, perhaps for people with disabilities, is on several drawing boards. It is of a kind with the sexual analogue of tele-health, "teledildonics," a potentially rich source of ethical issues best mooted elsewhere.

8 Biomedical research, from genomes to populations
Big Data and the growth of knowledge

As health information becomes voluminous and ubiquitous, an individual's right to control it is most usefully framed as a function of informed or valid consent. Balancing privacy and the benefits of using others' health information is one of the most interesting and difficult problems faced in a cloudy Big Data ecosystem in the digital health universe. In this chapter we challenge customary distinctions among clinical, research, and public health data, as well as the notion of "secondary use"; promote solidarity as a counterweight to autonomy and emphasize the willingness of many people to contribute their information to science; mull the role of community engagement, "citizen science," and the use of social media and other data sources; identify issues in bioinformatics and data mining; and conclude with a review of translational science and its advancement of trusted governance as a social and ethical partner in biomedical inquiry.

Ethics, wrongdoing, and best practices

Biomedical research saves, improves, and enriches human lives. We are better today for it, and will be better in the future because of it, most likely.

The conduct of biomedical research is, now, computational. Data and information are sought, found, saved, analyzed, shared, and, sometimes, transmuted into knowledge with the help of computers. It could not be otherwise – not anymore. We study cancer and backache, aberrant behavior and head-colds, heart disease and infectious disease with a computer being used at many points in the research. Scientists study maladies we get from living with each other and from aging; from work, injury, and sex; and our genes can make us sick. It is an information-intensive enterprise, and the tools of information technology are not only essential to the process but also shape it, sometimes in ways about which we know little.

The intersection of ethics, computing, and biomedical research is rich and complex, overwhelmingly because the data and information we study are about people. The issues of greatest interest for us are how – by what light and by what right – we ought to acquire, analyze, and use what we discover. Some of the issues we face here are related to standard components of the research ethics curriculum: valid consent, privacy, acceptable risk, vulnerable populations, and so on. Others are creatures of our computational wherewithal, especially the power of information technology to collect and analyze vast amounts of data such that well-known rules about consent and privacy do not clearly apply.

We have an opportunity to remind colleagues of something that is so obvious we sometimes forget it: The insights and requirements identified by ethical inquiry precede the rules of law. That is, recalling the discussion from Chapter 6, legislatures and parliaments would not know what to require or forbid if they did not have some grounding in what is antecedently identified to be permissible or impermissible. Determining what is right and wrong must come before determining what is legal and illegal. We have tended, understandably, to focus on wrongdoing. This is in part because the history of human-subject research includes cases of grievous and intentional mistakes at the dawn of modern biomedical research. The middle of the twentieth century saw wartime death-camp experiments in Europe and Asia and terrible abuses of vulnerable people in the Americas. The atrocities addressed by research ethics rules initially emerging from Nuremberg and Tuskegee demanded precisely such official rules (cf. Kass et al. 2013). Although we do not know what similar outrages these rules have prevented, we might be permitted to infer they have protected many people from harms and wrongs that might have been caused and done in the service of science.

Writing those rules was in some respects easy: There is nothing ethically *interesting* about Nazi hypothermia experiments or withholding syphilis treatment from a minority population in Alabama. The wrongness of that kind of research can be articulated straightforwardly,[1] and we have tried to do so for generations of horrified students. Much the same is true for that part of the research ethics curriculum that trumpets indignation over fabrication, falsification, and plagiarism, most instances of which are clearly illicit. It is not that students should not learn something about the history of human-subject research or the standards for data management and publication. Rather, our curricula will do better to emphasize best practices to be emulated, thoughtfulness about social responsibility in the conduct of research, and what the US Presidential Commission for the Study of Bioethical Issues (2011) called the importance of researchers to continue fostering the "earned confidence" of the citizens, who pay for much of their research in the first place. Hence, what is wanted now is a curriculum that emphasizes not atrocity, plagiarism, torture, and other wrongdoing, but research integrity with examples that celebrate good practice. This is nicely put by Mark Yarborough and Lawrence Hunter in "Teaching research ethics better: focus on excellent science, not bad scientists":

> Mandated instructional activities typically focus heavily on avoiding plagiarism, falsifying data, wrongly assigning authorship, and the like. While there may be a need at times to address such professional lapses in ethics learning, to make them the principal focus of what is too often, at least at the graduate and postgraduate level, the entirety of ethics learning in a science curriculum can have very negative consequences for many learners. Learners may find such courses peripheral to their interests, or even a distraction from what they consider their "real work" to be, meaning that the opportunity for effective education in ethics is largely lost when the thrust of a RCR course is avoiding misbehavior and other deviations from professional norms.
>
> (Yarborough and Hunter 2013, 201; citing Baldwin et al. 1991; cf. Yarborough 2014)

It is at the least difficult and probably impossible to document instances of research wrongdoing that did *not* occur because of good education. A similar challenge awaits anyone seeking to measure the amount, degree, or magnitude of public trust in science, and whether it has changed and, if so, why. It has been reported that the oft-invoked "Tuskegee legacy," that is, the idea that contemporary African Americans distrust biomedical research because of the syphilis experiment, is baseless (Katz et al. 2008). There is some evidence that distrust of science is related to political ideology (Gauchat 2012; Lewandowsky et al. 2013), though this is more in relation to issues such as genetically modified organisms, climate change, and vaccination. Research is haphazardly shared with citizens through the news and other popular media, museums, and word of mouth, and it is not obvious how much the (perceived) behavior of scientists or their treatment of people and animals in research affects feelings of trust. It could profitably be hypothesized that actual and perceived conflicts of interest are a greater source of mistrust, given the world's third-of-a-trillion-dollar biomedical research budget[2] and news reports about entrepreneurial science (Kraemer Diaz et al. 2015; Perry et al. 2014).

Biomedical informatics has blossomed as a discipline and changed the research ethics fabric. In what follows, three issues will be considered: data and Big Data analysis, including the proper roles of consent and privacy; bioinformatics, or the use of computational tools to manage and analyze genetic and genomic data; and public health informatics, or the creation and use of population-based data resources. If biomedical research is to continue to thrive, we need a better view of the computational threads running through that fabric.

Data ethics and biomedical science

Distinctions can increase conceptual clarity and advance explanation and understanding. Depending on what is being distinguished from what, the effort to provide such illumination can be dependent on context and so must be open to revision as the world changes. This is the case with the concept of "biomedical data." We have traditionally distinguished among three types or zones of data capture:

- clinical data, or that captured during interactions between patients and health professionals or patients and various instruments and tests
- research data, or that acquired during scientific studies or observations
- public health data, that is, data generated by population-based assays, surveys, geographic information systems, and so on

These distinctions once served us well, for the most part, pointing to places where privacy or consent needed attention. This is no longer the case (Kass et al. 2013). Rather than guide or instruct, these distinctions, often inscribed in law, institutional policy, and daily practice, have become artifacts of a time when the three zones were almost always distinct, separate, and disconnected. Clinical data did not become research data or public health data absent a focused effort to make it so, often at no small effort or expense. Overwhelmingly most of what was observed, recorded, or measured in the practice or hospital was sequestered in the isolated patient record, or lost. Research data and public health data were not available in clinical contexts before publication, and even then we did a poor job of it. The growth of the global research enterprise in the twentieth century made this a damnable shortcoming. That there was so much research—most of it unknown or inaccessible to clinicians—was correctly recognized by the epidemiologist Archie Cochrane as a collective methodological failure: "It is surely a great criticism of our profession that we have not organised a critical summary, by specialty or subspecialty, adapted periodically, of all relevant randomized controlled trials" (Cochrane 1979).

This is one of the foundations of what we have come to call "evidence-based medicine" or more broadly "evidence-based practice." Originally an insight about data synthesis by Thomas Beddoes (1760–1808) and Pierre Charles Alexandre Louis (1787–1872), the need for some reliable way to render a riot of data and information useful for clinicians has itself been framed as an ethical imperative (Goodman 2003; and recall the discussion from

Chapter 1). That it also engendered passionate opposition from some clinicians and philosophers should be understood to represent well-motivated attempts to improve what should be, and is otherwise, unavoidable – the need to do a better job putting the fruits of research on the table of clinical practice. At that level of abstraction there is surely no good reason to oppose it. In any case, what evidence-based practice requires is a reliable and nimble means of fueling the epistemic engine that takes data and information and turns them into knowledge that reduces suffering and prolongs life.

This is an information-intensive undertaking, and it lays bare a great cycle of empirical inquiry. If every clinical encounter generates data and information, can there be a reason, any *good* reason, not to use that information for the sake of other patients? Listen to the historian Roy Porter, quoting and commenting on Beddoes's 1808 "Letter to the Right Honourable Sir Joseph Banks … on the Causes and Removal of the Prevailing Discontents, Imperfections, and Abuses, in Medicine":

> Beddoes proposed two solutions. First, systematic collection and indexing of medical facts. "Why should not reports be transmitted at fixed periods from all the hospitals and medical charities in the kingdom to a central board?" Other "charitable establishments for the relief of the indigent sick" must also supply information, as should physicians at large. Data should be processed by a paid clerical staff, and made freely available. Seminars should be held. The stimulus to comparison and criticisms would sift good practice from bad. "What would be the effect", Beddoes mused, of "register offices, not exactly for receiving votive tablets, like certain ancient temples, but in which attestations, both of the good and of the evil, that appears to be done by practitioners of medicine, should be deposited?" Without effective information storage, retrieval and dissemination, medicine would never take its place amongst the progressive sciences. "To lose a single fact may be to lose many lives. Yet ten thousand, perhaps, are lost for one that is preserved; and all for want of a system among our theatres of disease, combined with the establishment of a national bank of medical wealth, where each individual practitioner may deposit his grains of knowledge, and draw out, in return, the stock, accumulated by all his brethren". … Second, to complement his medical bank, Beddoes urged his fellows to publish more…
>
> (Porter 1992, 10, notes omitted; this passage is quoted by Goodman 2003, 4)[3]

Imagine a nurse or physician who on Monday learned something interesting while caring for a patient. Then, on Friday, the same physician realized that what she learned on Monday might be useful in the care of a different patient. Is there anywhere in the world a privacy advocate so silly and bold as to suggest that using information from the first patient to care for the second patient was impermissible or illicit, perhaps as an affront to confidentiality? Is there an ethics boffin so pure and uncompromising as to argue that such a secondary use requires the informed consent of the first patient? This is the paradigm case of "secondary use," a use which has shaped, guided, and informed clinical practice for millennia. To suggest or even hint that such use poses challenges for privacy or consent is fundamentally to miss the point of wise and attentive clinical practice and, indeed, the core insight underlying what we now call "learning health care systems." Here is how I once put it:

> Consider a hypothetical physician who refused to incorporate years of experience when making future clinical judgments because to do so would mean using information about prior patients without their explicit permission. We would regard such a physician as unfit for practice – the very idea that one would decline to learn from experience (and cite patient privacy preferences in the process) would be medically and morally fatuous and kooky.

Moreover, any patient who insisted her physician or nurse not apply insights from her case to future patients would be no less peculiar. It would be equally and ethically bizarre if the patient cited a right to privacy, that is, suggested that such a subsequent use of her personal information would constitute a violation of her confidentiality. If, on the other hand, the clinician were to tell the subsequent patient that her case was just like that of Ms. Crabtree of 123 Elm Street, then such a disclosure would constitute an unacceptable violation. (Goodman 2010, 61)

In clinical practice, the grain or datum that merges with others to become data, and, eventually, Big Data, is a grain whose use is not merely permissible – it is morally obligatory. Failure to use and leverage these data shows no great respect for privacy and constitutes no homage to the tenets of valid consent. It is an ethical failure, a mistake. Beddoes might or might not have been hyperbolic in holding that "To lose a single fact may be to lose many lives," but the larger point is not open to dispute: Facts do save lives. If, as we saw in Chapter 3, privacy is both precious but not absolute, we must begin to frame the data-use versus data-privacy debate in such a way as to sacrifice neither to the other.

We have been talking about clinical data, or, as noted above, "that captured during interactions between patients and health professionals or patients and various instruments and tests." While an individual clinician might make good use of idiosyncratic or episodic connections between or among data, such serendipity relies on luck as much as on thoughtful analysis. If, as alleged, there is a moral imperative to use such good fortune in the care of patients, the imperative expands with the availability of data. We must, that is, not await the next fortuitous observation in hopes it will improve patient care but, rather, set about marshaling that data to improve the health of patients and, indeed, of populations. We now have the ability to coordinate large-scale data capture and analysis in electronic health records. This means that in the evolution of data collection and management, "the next step is to transform healthcare big data into actionable knowledge" (Ross et al. 2014, 97; cf. Buguski et al. 2009 for the hope of more robust postmarket surveillance and a "new kind of pharmacovigilance" ... to "detect, assess, and understand beneficial drug side effects [or expanded drug interactions] that may become apparent during their development or use"; and Szczepaniak et al. 2006 for the role of ubiquitous monitoring for early detection of public health emergencies).

Patient data (clinical data, electronic health record data) constitute a third of our "great cycle of empirical inquiry." We already have mastered the task of analyzing these data via the "retrospective chart review." Most jurisdictions permit such reviews after assessment by institutional review boards or research ethics committees; however, the consent of individuals is not needed – nor should it be. Consider that we have, for better or worse, drawn a distinction between quality assessment, which good institutions undertake to improve practice, and chart reviews, which are regarded as human-subject research. The former are universally regarded as uncontroversial and require no special permission; it would be irresponsible not to conduct such assessments. But as soon as the role of the data analyzer shifts from administrator to investigator, everything changes. There are several reasons for this, but paramount is likely to be the definition of "research" as adopted in US law and adapted in Europe and elsewhere. Research, according to the US Code of Federal Regulations, is "a systematic investigation, including research development, testing and evaluation, designed to develop or contribute to generalizable knowledge."[4] This captures the intuition that data and information applicable only to one institution, for instance, are not "generalizable" or generally applicable to others.

It is not *ethically* clear why a systematic chart review by a researcher should enjoy greater protection or scrutiny than an otherwise indistinguishable systematic chart review by administrators; one might even argue that because the former will be shared with others and so perhaps improve quality at other institutions as well, it should be encouraged – and it is the administrative use of patient data that should be regulated. Because intentions matter in ethics, suppose that the administrative use of patient data is intended to reduce costs by justifying the limitation of certain interventions. Is that more or less praiseworthy or blameworthy than using patient data to improve the health of all patients similarly treated everywhere?

Moreover, the traditional chart review conjures images of an administrator or a researcher sitting at a table filled with heaps of paper binders filling "in" and "out" baskets. In fact, we now have query tools to automate these reviews, database search engines to tune the queries, and data mining algorithms to wring as much useful data, if not information, as possible from collections of patient information.[5] Significantly, these search tools can automatically de-identify patient data, occulting from administrators or researchers data or information that would otherwise make it easy to pick out, recognize, or identify an individual. That is, information technology tools may on occasion be regarded as tools to protect confidentiality.

Indeed, most biomedical research does not consist in sifting through existing patient data, but in generating more of it, namely through clinical trials. The first controlled clinical trial apparently took place in 1944, when the British Medical Research Council studied the effects of the antibiotic patulin (a mycotoxin produced by *Penicillium* and other molds and found in apples and other foods) on the common cold. It didn't work, but it inaugurated the age of the clinical trial (Chalmers and Clarke 2004).[6] The US National Institutes of Health's clinicaltrials.gov Web site in 2015 listed nearly 185,000 ongoing studies in 188 countries, including the United States; the European Medicines Agency's www.clinicaltrialsregister.eu listed about 25,000. Those trials represent a lot of patient data, much of it documented in the participants' medical records. Should these data, in an electronic health record, for instance, and whether or not noted or acted upon by clinicians, be regarded exclusively as research data?

Public health informatics and the fallacy of "secondary use"

The discussion so far should make clear that the distinction between "clinical data" and "research data" is neither accurate nor, in consequence, useful. If patient data and information are routinely collected and stored in electronic health records, then the ease with which such data and information can be analyzed should be understood to entail an obligation to conduct such analyses. I have argued throughout that electronic tools actually and often arrive with correlate duties to use them wisely, and that the customary "dilemma savoring" we scorned in Chapter 3 continues to serve us poorly. Clinical data *ought* to become research data. Put differently, and assuming governance systems that honor the trust of ordinary people in the biomedical research enterprise, there are no detectable good arguments to enjoin the use of clinical data *as* research data or to discourage the creation of registries to facilitate that use. This argument grows stronger when we make clear that its scope includes the health of populations.

The histories of epidemiology and public health are histories of increasingly refined efforts by (generally) trustworthy scientists to identify data patterns and determine if these patterns reveal causal connections, and, if so, to use these insights to improve the health of communities. It would be irresponsible not to do so (Goodman and Meslin 2014).

From ancient pattern-seekers such as Hippocrates[7] through medieval observers such as Paracelsus and early modern epidemiologists such as John Snow, to contemporary syndromic surveillance trackers, it would be (perhaps literally) unthinkable to suggest that their work should be forbidden because their use of data about people was not based on the permission of each of them, or as mysterious, preceded by an effort to obtain such permission. A favorite example is the evolution of automobile safety seats for children. Years of systematic analysis of injuries and deaths caused by a lack of child restraints, tuned by years of systematic analysis of misuse of such restraints, have led to the development of generally reliable automobile restraints for children. In several countries, analyses of hospital records, police notes, emergency medical technician reports, and other resources – none of it with any consent whatsoever – have led to protection measures that save thousands of lives annually (see, e.g., Howard 2002; Yakupcin 2005). Is there anyone anywhere who would seriously suggest that such analyses were impermissible, illicit, or unethical? Would anyone not attempting parody actually seek to impose a consent requirement for such analysis in the future?

Crowdsourcing, "citizen science," and Web queries

As we saw in Chapter 7, many people do not need to be won over; they actually go out of their way to make their health data and information available. In crowdsourcing, people make themselves available and respond to requests for their information. "Participatory health initiatives" are in some sense a public demand for engagement with investigators as "an asset to medical discovery" (Swan 2012b). It is likely that those with the greatest zeal for this effort are patients, that is, people who are sick and want not to be. As my friend and colleague Richard Bookman has beautifully expressed it, "Healthy people want more privacy; sick people want more research."[8]

This insight becomes an inclination, a disposition to share. It is perhaps a desire to create and live in a scientifico-social commons. It is not a rejection of government and institutional privacy protections as much as a desire to anticipate them, in part by front-loading consent. It gets better. Maybe even healthy people want to contribute. In "The Resilience Project" led by Icahn School of Medicine at Mount Sinai in New York and Sage Bionetworks, "You can donate your DNA to medical research as we search for 'healthy' adults who have rare genetic changes that we'd expect to cause severe illness in childhood. We know that these 'resilient' people exist, and we believe if we can understand what is protecting them from illness, then we can make advances towards treating or even preventing these diseases."[9] Secondary mutations can have a protective effect against genetically caused or mediated maladies, and with enough analysis of enough DNA samples, there is hope that we will be able to shift focus from curing these maladies to preventing them; studies of healthy people have identified mutations related to the prevention of HIV infection, modification of sickle-cell disease, and prevention of cardiovascular disease (Friend and Schadt 2014). The project obviously requires the cooperation of healthy people; 1 million volunteers are sought. Why would healthy persons donate their DNA? That is, "What would be their motivation? Low risk and potentially high reward. Enabling participants to assess whether they can serve as an 'unexpected hero' to others who are afflicted with catastrophic disease could be personally inspiring" (ibid., 971).

John Wilbanks, also of Sage Bionetworks, has developed a "Portable Legal Consent" to capture the finding that "the overwhelming response has been not a desire for differential consent that allows only academic use, or a consent only for a certain field of use; instead, participants are far more concerned about the *kind of data* they have and how they would like to donate it" (Wilbanks 2014, 248, original emphasis). Refining this, studying it, getting it right establishes a platform for exciting future work in genetics. The value and utility of "citizen science," or a kind of deputization of nonscientists to participate in an empirical inquiry, has been and is being demonstrated in cosmology, environmental studies, biology, and elsewhere. It is ripe for Big Data collection and analysis (Hochachka et al. 2012), and its usefulness in human health is inchoate. This means that citizen science itself needs more research, research governed by the kinds of ethical beacons discussed in Chapter 4.

The point, made in several places in this book, sometimes tacitly, is that there are many ethical questions whose answers are likely to depend on additional empirical work; some of that work will be on research methods, some on patient preferences, and some on the scope, utility, and impediments of informed or valid consent. This stance is not to succumb to the "is/ought" or naturalistic fallacy, in which identifying a good depends on "natural" properties. It is, rather, to acknowledge that for utilitarian and other ethics, a better and deeper understanding can be shaped by more evidence about how the world works, and what kinds of consequences can be expected from different actions and policies; indeed, this is in part why so much emphasis is placed in this chapter in trying to identify the scope and depth of people's willingness to contribute their data and information (including that contained in biological materials) for research.

If "voluntary" means something like "with or of free choice," "involuntary" means "against one's will," and "nonvoluntary" entails "without having been asked" – a not-uncommon plural distinction – then in addition to crowdsourcing and citizen science, we should have a look at the scope and reliability of nonvoluntary citizen science, namely the analysis of Web browser searches to support inferences about public health, including outbreaks of dangerous diseases (Brownstein et al. 2009). Social networking services, Web queries, and even Wikipedia page views have been used to study influenza transmission (Hiller et al. 2013; Salathé et al. 2013,) as well as food-borne illnesses, HIV, dengue, tuberculosis, and others. The results are mixed, but suggestive.

Two primary ethical issues are of interest here. One is shaped by the question whether surveillance of online behavior is intrusive or constitutes some sort of invasion of privacy. It is difficult to generate too much concern on this account: The owners of Web browsers have never suggested, offered, or promised that search strings sent to another computer or server were privileged or protected in the way we are discussing. The permissibility of any tracking or collection will need to be a function of who is doing the monitoring and for what purpose. An academic or government epidemiologist tracking searches to improve pandemic influenza predictions will enjoy ethical warrant superior to that of a financial services firm monitoring the clickstream in hopes of being able to identify minority communities against which to discriminate. It has also become commonplace to observe that the conditions for using many tools include consent to allow the monitoring of their use and that the value of convenience customarily supersedes worries about surveillance, monitoring, or privacy. It is also likely that many would prefer no such trade-off but have resigned themselves to the intrusion. In any case, if, as seems to be equally commonplace, Web users have resigned themselves to tracking by credit card firms, banks, and all manner of commerce, then it is difficult to sound much of an alarm over tracking to improve public health.

Second, we should inquire after what should evolve to be best standards in online public health surveillance.[10] Although it is still too early to be clear about such standards, a good start is in the criteria for responsible conduct of research we surveyed in Chapter 4 – standards to which we will return again later in discussing ethics in bioinformatics. Cast as duties, *transparency, veracity, and accountability/responsibility* should be seen to have just such a large a role in online surveillance as in the laboratory. Indeed, in a better world, these duties would have been embraced by all professionals in all enterprises – not just scientists.

Autonomy, solidarity, and "presumed solidarity"

As was observed at the beginning of this chapter, many of the well-motivated rules under which we conduct human-subject research were shaped by atrocities in Alabama and in European concentration camps. Because of the special sensitivity of health information, post-Tuskegee legislators were wise to include protection of such information, though one may be forgiven for speculating that if the worst thing the Nazis or Public Health Service investigators did was violate confidentiality, we would be living under entirely different regulatory structures. Neither the 1979 Belmont Report,[11] which undergirds all subsequent US human-subject-protection law, nor the postwar Nuremberg Code,[12] mentions privacy, confidentiality, or any need to require consent to permit data use. What the Belmont Report does is enshrine "respect for persons" and its two-component "moral requirements: the requirement to acknowledge autonomy and the requirement to protect those with diminished autonomy."[13]

This celebration of autonomy, or self-determination, is, since Kant, a staple of Western moral philosophy – as are attempts to identify its limits. Philosophers, perhaps especially Jürgen Habermas, struggled with balancing autonomy and solidarity, which likewise enjoys a preeminent role. In bioethics and other applied ethics, however, there is a significant bifurcation of emphasis between European and American approaches. Albert R. Jonsen (one of the members of the National Commission for the Protection of Human Subjects of Biomedical and Behavioral Research, which produced the Belmont Report) explains that "The ideal of solidarity, the communal responsibility to help those in need, has religious and socialist roots that pervade bioethical thinking across Europe. Solidarity is a European bioethical principle that has only a weak reflection in the American principle of justice" (Jonsen 1998, 379). In Canada, a key report during the SARS crisis assigned a central role to solidarity (University of Toronto Joint Centre for Bioethics 2005).

The tension here is at the very core of our attempt to find a balance between the duty to protect data (and so respect the autonomy of those whom the data pertain to) and the duty to contribute to the common good, especially when doing so requires no effort whatsoever (and so respect the positive human inclination to solidarity, to help others). Addressing, let alone resolving or eliminating, this tension is complex and tricky. We all enjoy and even depend on our autonomy, and respecting it engenders trust – but we also depend on public health services, which, in turn, depend on solidarity. This means we must be careful lest the heavy-handed playing of a solidarity trump card does something to erode that trust.

Fortunately, most Western public health agencies seem to enjoy the trust of the populations they serve. How else can we explain the absence of credible objection to the computational maintenance of vital statistics, countless disease registries, vaccine records, poison-control data sets, vastly many health surveillance projects, and so on, and on? Most of us actually assume and depend on these services, usually without moral consternation about abridgments of our autonomy. We are indifferent to the use of information technology to constitute and study these repositories (as if any of them, anymore, could be maintained on paper). Indeed, the extraordinary success of the public health enterprise, with millions, perhaps billions, of lives improved, if not saved, provides powerful utilitarian warrant for the kind of "presumed solidarity" being mooted here. For instance:

> For more than three decades, the state government of Western Australia has been collecting one of the world's largest administrative health datasets, including birth records, midwives' notifications, cancer registrations, inpatient hospital morbidity, in-patient and public out-patient, mental health services data and death records. Used in combination with medical record audits, the WA dataset provides a platform for comprehensive evaluation of health system performance. Moreover, investigators have developed a system for linkage that is aimed at meeting the dual goals of protecting privacy and enabling health systems research. This "win-win" approach results from keeping any identifiable information from the researchers, who only need the linked data on exposures and outcomes for their analyses. Of note, since this program has been in place, general requests for access to identifiable data have declined markedly. Indeed, when officials asked people in the general community if they approved of their information being used in this way, they found that citizens were not only supportive of the use, but they questioned why it was not already in use for research purposes.   (Meslin and Goodman 2010; cf. Marquard and Brennan 2009)[14]

In addition:

> Many studies noted participants' lack of knowledge about research processes and existing safeguards and this was reflected in the focus groups. Focus group participants became more accepting of the use of pre-collected medical data without consent after being given information about selection bias and research processes. All participants were keen to contribute to NHS-related research but some were concerned about data-sharing for commercial gain and the potential misuse of information. Increasing public education about research and specific targeted information provision could promote trust in research processes and safeguards, which in turn could increase the acceptability of research without specific consent where the need for consent would lead to biased findings and impede research necessary to improve public health.   (Hill et al. 2013)

Further:

> what our participants care about most is the specific purpose for using information, and among the choices we investigated, the goal they most privilege is research ... To our surprise, the sensitivity of the health information – at least within the range we presented (personal medical history plus personal genetic test results vs. personal medical history alone) – was not important. This finding contrasts with the notion that patients view genetic information as particularly sensitive. It may add support to the arguments against privileging genetic information, as some experts have argued ... Relationships with the health care system are associated with support for sharing health information. Participants with high levels of distrust of the health care system, those without a usual source of care, and those who had recently experienced cost barriers to care were less supportive of secondary uses.

> (Grande et al. 2013, 1802, notes omitted; cf. Grande et al. 2014)

But now this, both to sound a cautionary note and to suggest that although citizens might be divided on their enthusiasm for sharing data, any reluctance can be difficult to understand:

> People are known for making decisions which in many cases subvert their interests. Consumer psychology research has for instance shown that people happily accept "default" positions such that if one asks if someone wants or values something, the number of respondents who agree is smaller than if respondents are asked to "opt out" or decline to disagree. This insight, were it applied more widely in organ procurement, for example, which most people find inoffensive, would save thousands of lives. What Max H. Bazerman and colleagues have called the "irrational preference for harms of omission over harms of action" has yet to be explored in the context of privacy and secondary-use preferences regarding the use of personal data for public health.
>
> (Goodman 2010, 62; citing Baron 1998 and Johnson and Goldstein 2003; and quoting Moore et al. 2006)

Moreover, this continues:

> Hypotheses therefore to be tested explicitly … include that ordinary patients, all things being equal:
>
> 1. would not object to the use of their information for public health;
> 2. assume such use is already occurring; and
> 3. agree they have a moral obligation to permit such use.

Here are some lessons to draw: Generally, people want to support research, especially by trusted entities; they at least sometimes, perhaps often, assume that their personal information is already being used without their explicit permission and for the purpose of helping others, and so they do not object; they prefer research that is not commercially motivated; they sometimes act against their own interests; they like to be asked about the use of their information and data. This is apparently and especially true for biobanks. A European survey found less concern about privacy than about the ability to control the use of data and information in biological material (Snell et al. 2012). But such control should be on the list of informatics deliverables. Future electronic health records and biorepositories will enable more-or-less fine-grained electronic control of subsequent use by the people who are the sources of the information (Eder et al. 2012; and see the collection by Häyry et al. 2007 for a number of helpful analyses; recall, moreover, the discussion of granular patient control over data use in Chapter 1). The satisfaction and comfort of that control might alone be enough to generate cohorts of the sizes needed for credible research. Come the day when all biobanks are digital, indeed, it will make no sense whatever to draw blood or take a buccal swab, sequence a patient's genome, curate the digital result, render it machine tractable, and then give the patient a piece of paper to sign. It might be asked why we are making it difficult for them to help.

We have, nevertheless and somehow, created an industry of risk savoring based on the presumption that we need to protect ordinary citizens from people who are trying to improve their health, if not save their lives (and if they are indifferent about that, their neighbors' lives).[15] In fact, the risk of many kinds of computational analysis is quite low, and it has been compellingly argued that comparative effectiveness research, for instance, is a good example of a type of systematic inquiry for which consent is not necessary (Gostin et al. 2001). Who on campus, at the hospital, or in the clinic has not heard that the reason we need strict privacy rules is to protect us from public humiliation, erosion of social benefits, and the loss of income or employment? But that is the wrong direction in advocating for privacy and confidentiality protections. Rather, abuse of data by insurance companies and employers should locate the moral center of our need for rules and policies, not the efforts by scientists and administrators who are trying to analyze our de-identified data in very large data warehouses. Laws against discrimination and strict penalties for inappropriate use take us in the right direction as regards our greatest fears. In the United States, the 2010 Affordable Care Act's elimination of "pre-existing conditions" is precisely what was necessary to address risk and fear of discrimination by insurers and employers. That said, the reason we do want strict privacy rules is to protect a right, independently of the consequences of its violation. That right, to privacy, is precious but, as discussed throughout here, must also be balanced against the benefits to be gained by trusted agents doing innovative research to improve the health of individuals and communities.

It has been suggested that we have framed our concerns backwards and that, perhaps, "health care institutions have unwittingly inverted the question that needs answering. Rather than 'Why risk alarming our patients by using their health care data for research?' perhaps we should be asking, 'Why is our first obligation not to ensure that our patients' data are used for research as they wish and expect them to be used?'" (Kohane 2013, 1807). It is as if, perhaps, we have grounds not merely to presume consent, with appropriate safeguards, but to regard it, in one fashion or another, as a kind of "latent consent" which we have at least some warrant to rely on.[16] From the Western Australia data set to the US Food and Drug Administration's Sentinel and Mini-Sentinel projects[17] to the Centers for Disease Control and Prevention's National Program of Cancer Registries (and assorted software tools) to the UK's National Health Service Central Register to the European Commission's rare diseases registries to the World Health Organization's Global Public Health Intelligence Network, the systematic collection and analysis of data about people for the health of populations is a grand and tacit recognition and embodiment of the duties that attach to solidarity.

The computational (or, indeed, any) use of aggregated personal health data and information in these "collaboratories" is, moreover, an easy way for citizens to express solidarity. As above, it requires no effort, costs them nothing, and entails vanishingly small risk. If there were a way to "opt out" or refuse to permit one's data or information to be thus stored and analyzed, it would bias if not corrupt the datasets and, in any case, render them less effective in preventing disease and other misfortune. Anyone who wants to opt out therefore emerges as parallel to vaccine "free riders," or those who refuse to vaccinate their children while benefiting from the herd immunity conferred on those who do, or those who refrain from being organ donors even though they would gladly accept another's donated kidney, liver, or heart if failing to do so meant dying. These are not homages to or celebrations of autonomy, not actualized self-determination, not brave assertions of individual rights against the oppressive designs of government epidemiologists. They are, instead, a form of cheating or gaming the system. Here, however, is the correct stance:

> In the context of popular belief in the primacy of autonomy, much has been written about the need to use health data generally to support the claim that governments and other health care providing institutions are morally obligated to provide the most effective and efficient care to the greatest number of citizens possible. This collection and use of data requires that the public participate, and public participation requires public trust ...

> Scientists and clinicians cannot maximize public health or clinical benefits without access to public health data, and access to those data depends on the public's trust that they are protected from both rogue access and inappropriate use. The secure space for private information to be used for public good is provided by policies that constrain the use of data to those purposes for which they were intended and protect data from unauthorized access. (Lee 2014, 49; cf. Bayer and Fairchild 2002; Lee et al. 2012; Rubel 2012)

These constraints, laid out by Lee and Gostin (2009), include collecting data only for legitimate purposes, having strong security measures in place, disseminating data to relevant stakeholders, and ensuring that all who have access to data are responsible stewards. These are precisely among the tools to be explored and developed as we try to maintain trust while presuming solidarity. This exploration and development will acquire increasing importance as our software improves and its reach widens. Any nontrivial failure in these efforts is likely to lead to exaggerated autonomy claims of the sort that undermine public health.

Indeed, as the clinical data versus research data distinction has been found to be unhelpful, it should perhaps now be clear that the third main data source identified earlier, that is, public health data, is, as such, also not illuminating in a plurally interconnected world. In the same way that we try to educate physicians and nurses about their important roles as frontline agents and actors in protecting the health of populations, it also makes sense to use their data.

The excitement to do that is palpable: "Clinical research is on the threshold of a new era in which electronic health records ... are gaining an important novel supporting role," writes one team exploring security and privacy as an integral part of the research enterprise (Coorevits et al. 2013, 547). Addressing one of the largest challenges facing clinical trial investigators, that effort has produced "a protocol feasibility prototype which is used for finding patients eligible for clinical trials from multiple sources." Another team that worked on policy issues declared early in the era of Big Data that "Secondary uses of health data can enhance individuals' health care experiences, expand knowledge about diseases and treatments, strengthen understanding of health care systems' effectiveness and efficiency, support public health and security goals, and aid businesses in meeting customers' needs" (Safran et al. 2007, 2).

Health data networks are expanding our understanding of the utility of large-scale data capture (Curtis et al. 2014). One such is "ESPnet," an open-source system developed by Harvard Medical School's Department of Population Medicine:

> [This] is a disease surveillance software application that can extract and analyze data from electronic health record systems for events of public health importance [and] a software application that enables controlled, secure, distributed analyses of health data owned by different organizations and stored in different locations. ... Combining these two technologies allows hospitals and clinics to give health departments controlled access to their EHR data monitor health indicators in their patient populations and makes it possible for health departments to easily query the EHR systems of multiple providers at once to get a population level view of health indicators. ... ESPnet also supports an intelligent presentation system, the RiskScape, which graphically displays population level surveillance data to inform public health ... Hospitals and clinics retain full control over their data at all times. ESPnet runs behind the host practice's firewall and only permits external users to run analyses and/or retrieve data that have been approved by the hospital or clinic.[18]

Significantly, once we cross-train physicians and researchers to attend to the needs of public health, and, presumably, public health workers to do the same for their counterparts, we further undermine the notion that any datum belongs to any particular purpose. A hospital-based infectious disease report might be used for an individual patient, but surely it should also and immediately be regarded as having utility for anyone doing hospital epidemiology or community disease mapping and tracking. Or consider the many routine hospital tests conducted for individual patients, many of which are barely noted and then stored. It could very well be the case that the first actual use of these data will be only after they are aggregated and analyzed for a community or population. Once this is so, then, what is the *primary use* of the data? This is no idle question, and its answer is important not just for conceptual clarity but also because we have made so very much of what it means to be a *secondary use* of data. We should pause here briefly.[19]

We have in place a vast skein of well-motivated rules governing the collection and use of most clinical and research data. In Chapter 3 we reviewed many of the underpinnings, some ancient, of privacy rules. While most patients and research subjects likely are as well informed about these rules as about their foundations or, say, in the United States, the Common Rule governing human-subject research, there is a large, collective understanding that some sort of rules are in place. We for the most part reckon when we consent to treatment or to participate in research that our personal information will be safeguarded – more or less; this is an explicit requirement of most research consent forms, if not processes. But the use of patient or participant data and information afterwards is traditionally a kind of terra incognita, unexplored, perilous. Absent those cases in which we strap on a reconsent requirement to "re-use" existing data, we have no particularly good rules to guide us in the ethics of such use. Remember "World Citizen 7s3j9t5p9r2m5y1z4" from Chapter 3? Suppose the fact that she was twice treated for a sexually transmitted infection in young adulthood was stored both in a networked general practice data repository and in a research data set; that is, the same fact. Reliable future security provisions prevent any evildoers from linking her name or other unique identifier to either of those two records. Is additional consent ethically required before:

- the District Public Health Agency can increase by 1 the number of women aged 20–30 treated twice for chlamydia in Ohio during that period?
- a statistician could perform a meta-analysis using aggregate data as published after the research survey?
- a practice guidelines working group could review the data to propose diagnostic best practices?

What we have come to call "secondary use" now emerges as a misnomer. It is a vague concept, imprecisely described or refined, and not effectively managed. If, as above, these data were collected with two primary intentions (clinical care and public health), then their use for public health cannot accurately be regarded as secondary at all. As the distinctions between and among data sources collapse – and, especially, as the people whose welfare is being protected acquire a deeper understanding of and appreciation for the ways their data and information are used and protected – there will be correspondingly diminished need to seek, repeatedly or continuously, their permission. Indeed, if this is right, they would not have it any other way. The successes of public health demonstrate this beautifully: Hundreds of years of behind-the-scenes data collection, health monitoring, and surveillance – all without explicit consent – have served us well and overwhelmingly without problem or rational protest. This is a good foundation on which to develop large-scale automated data capture and storage. What is required is a trusted and reliable system for smart, nuanced, and ethically optimized governance of large and complex computational health research projects.

Case study: social science tempest, Facebook teapot

If the social and behavioral sciences are to be of any use or interest, they must study humans in their native habitats. These have now come to include life and lives online. According to the Pew Internet Research Project, some three quarters (73%) of adults who access the Internet also use social networking sites; 71% use Facebook (Duggan and Smith 2013). This means, it could be argued, that the social science community would be irresponsible not to try to learn about the effects of Facebook on users, and vice versa.

The challenge here and, indeed, for much social science research, is how to provide adequate ethics review of such research in an environment governed by rules shaped, as we have seen, in the wake of biomedical research atrocities.

A study reported in the *Proceedings of the National Academy of Sciences* came to serve as a lens through which these challenges can be viewed. The study, of "emotional contagion," involved the manipulation of Facebook's "News Feed" to reduce the number of positive words and expressions to determine if that manipulation caused a corresponding reduction in positive posts (and increase in negative posts), and to reduce negative words and expressions to see if the opposite occurred (Kramer et al. 2014). Both interventions weakly confirmed that Facebook users reading sad news apparently became slightly sadder, and vice versa. That is, they found that emotional states can be altered and transferred among hundreds of thousands of Facebook users – that "emotions can spread throughout a network" without the awareness or knowledge of those whose moods were being tracked, or at least inferred.

This finding would be of far less interest were it not for the fact that mood disorders can help predict phenomena ranging from medical nonadherence to suicide. Still, what was studied here was not mood disorder but the ability of a social network to alter mood. Several facts bear on the ethical issues raised by the study.

First, Facebook at the time disclosed, albeit not prominently, that it might use member posts for "internal operations, including troubleshooting, data analysis, testing, research and service improvement."[20] The question here is whether this disclosure – that online behavior might be monitored or tracked for *research* – is adequate. After the episode, the policy was changed to say information will be used for "conducting academic research and surveys." In a cascading series of not-unreasonable assumptions, one may infer that most Internet inhabitants assume their behavior is being tracked and analyzed, and assume this is the case at least for business purposes. That, however, is not what is intended or understood by scientists, who are generally governed by laws (in the United States and Europe) drafted to protect participants in biomedical or social-behavioral science. While some measure of deception is permitted for studies of human behavior because disclosing the true purpose of the inquiry would confound the results, good practice normally requires a post-study debriefing

Second, the Facebook study was in fact reviewed by a US university's Institutional Review Board. The authors of the study reported to the journal that, "Because this experiment was conducted by Facebook, Inc. for internal purposes, the [IRB] determined that the project did not fall under [the institution's] Human Research Protection Program"; and that statement was confirmed by the university (Verma 2014). While US law applies to federally funded research, most institutions apply federal standards to all research as a matter of good practice. In the Facebook case and given the scientific goals of the study, it is clear that the research was not conducted merely or exclusively for internal Facebook business purposes. One can imagine a different IRB determination: one that required a more extensive and easy-to-access disclosure, an opportunity to opt out of such research studies, and a mechanism for public debriefing after the conclusion of the project.

Third, the study posed little or no risk to participants. While being a little sadder than would otherwise be the case is certainly a risk, we must be careful not to make too much of it. But the reasons for reviewing human-subject research (it is probably inaccurate to call data sources "participants" if they do not know they are being studied) include protecting subjects from both harms and wrongs. To the extent that (i) people prefer to know they are being studied and (ii) they are not so informed, then investigators might be said to have wronged them.

The Facebook Mood Manipulation Case engendered intense debate, online of course, in the informatics and bioethics communities. One of the most important points to emerge in both communities was this: While the individuals who were studied did not consent to being studied, such consent is not a universal requirement for ethical research. As we have seen throughout this chapter, there is a long and solid tradition and ample precedent for trusted organizations to analyze aggregated data in epidemiology, public health, health outcomes research, and so on. Such surveillance and analysis would be impossible if consent were required from each and every person whose data helped comprise the data set. Yet such surveillance and research saves lives, reduces error, and improves health care systems. It would be perverse to insist on fine-grained consent for such analyses – and worse to invoke "ethics" in the process.

Overstating the harm and wrong of the Facebook study risks imperiling the more important types of research we are duty-bound to conduct. That is, to draw any kind of parallel between a poorly reviewed study of whether some news stories make people sad and the kind of large-scale data analysis required for the success of learning health care systems is to endanger vital tools needed for the protection of individual patients and of entire populations. It would be very sad indeed if a group-pout on the Internet were to contribute to a civilization's distrust of the world's research mission.

Big Data ethics

If we could design a comprehensive health system from scratch, today, we might not create separate professions to undertake the tasks now expected of clinicians, researchers, and epidemiologists.[21] As we have tried to undermine the distinction among clinical, research, and public health data, we have also suggested that health professionals of all kinds should be able to generate, use, and analyze a range of data and information. This at any rate closes our "great cycle of empirical inquiry," an effort to justify the intentional collapsing of a longstanding distinction, and a consummation made possible by modern information technology, technology that is, and perhaps ought to be, agnostic as among the origins of its data.

This is "big data," really big data. At least as large, however, is our task of making sense of it to improve health. Perhaps larger still is the duty to ensure that as we do so, we retain the trust of those individual humans to whom the data pertain. Here is one grand but not implausible goal: to have a comprehensive web of data from research trials, genome analyses, clinical encounters, and public health surveillance, a kind of mega-, meta-, or uberverse, a vast data ecosystem with more grains than Beddoes could imagine, constantly growing and constantly challenging our ability to make sense of it. Efficient, and appropriate use, and "trust maintenance" may be the greatest ethical challenges posed by Big Data.[22]

The concepts of "appropriate use" and "appropriate users" advanced in Chapter 3 will guide us now. As we earlier suggested that online surveillance with the goal of discriminating against minorities would clearly be illicit, we can apply those distinctions here. The case of *Sorrell* v. *IMS Health Inc.* is instructive. In this case, the US Supreme Court in 2011 unfortunately struck down a Vermont law that "required data mining companies to obtain permission from individual providers before selling prescription records that included identifiable physician prescriber information to pharmaceutical companies for drug marketing" (Petersen et al. 2013, 35). It should be uncontroversial to assert that there are compelling ethical differences between such kinds of commercial monitoring and the kinds of science we are mulling here. Moreover, if it is true that ordinary people prefer their information be used for biomedical science and not marketing, then uses of the sort reviewed in *Sorrell* should be seen to be out of bounds. (Independently of the question whether the legal ruling was sound, this would be a case of a court making an ethical mistake.) It would be a damnable tragedy if such commercial data sniffing eroded public trust and if that erosion were to spill over to more ethically defensible bioscience inquiry.

Because Big Data could be so very big, we tend reflexively to assume that challenges it poses will be, well, bigger than those that arise from tiny data, mid-sized data, and so on. As to ethics, this is not necessarily clear. We long ago surpassed the ability of humans to analyze large data sets on paper, so it is legitimate to inquire whether really big data sets, or many of them interconnected, actually introduce new challenges. Any such challenges will be found in a zone plotted by large-scale data capture, and the trust-and-privacy challenges that raises; data mining software engineering; and therefore by the kinds of issues mooted in Chapter 4, on professionalism and data management.

One way to think about meeting these challenges, no matter their magnitude, is in the creative use of data access protocols and what has been called "privacy by design" (Khum and Ahalt 2013; recall also the discussion from Chapter 3). Where our current practice and regulatory structures regard data privacy as an accoutrement one attaches to uses of personal information, or a kind of procedural hat or scarf (think of consent requirements and study-by-study review), we might do better if we forged a process shaped by embedded and automated protections that wed access controls with smart and nimble data curation and processing to manage use and sharing (cf. Lane and Schur 2010).

Community engagement

Another positive move is patient and community engagement, which are essential for trust building and maintenance. If it is true that patients do not mind sharing their data but like to know they are doing so, then initiatives such as the Patient-Centered Outcomes Research Institute, created to support comparative effectiveness research, offer several means of both informing communities about research and encouraging "patients and other stakeholders to partner with researchers to study the issues that are most critical to them."[23] This has long been recognized as a duty of foreign researchers in low-middle-income countries (National Bioethics Advisory Commission 2001), but it is also good practice in all countries. This point is underscored by the Nuffield Council on Bioethics in a comprehensive report that reviews British "data initiatives in health systems," including the less-than-successful National Health Service's "care.data" program to capture clinical data in the Health and Social Care Information Centre, and the Scottish Informatics Programme, saluted for its "commitment to public engagement" (Nuffield Council on Bioethics 2015).[24]

This move – the leavening or imbuing of the research enterprise with community engagement – is of a piece with other efforts in practical ethics to address challenges when saying "no" hurts too much to be right or to make sense, when approaching issues with ultrafine granularity provides no structure and is only as good as the instant case, and when saying "yes" without adequate controls gives away precisely that which we hoped to accomplish: a reasoned method of ensuring that shared values become an integral part of the enterprise. When we get it right, we have made a significant contribution not only to applied ethics, but, as important, to public policy. Other examples of broadening the universe of ethical discourse and counsel to solve complex problems include efforts to manage financial conflicts of interest, rules to require special education for people whose work raises ethical issues, and requirements to establish review mechanisms to help ensure the protection of human subjects and research animals. (Rules for including community members on institutional review boards or research ethics committees represent a similar approach to including lay people in scientific undertakings.)

These tools or mechanisms are imperfect, and at many institutions they cause great consternation, if not hostility. ("I'd be making a lot more money if I weren't taking so much time with the online courses, if the conflict of interest committee wasn't so mean, and if the IRB wasn't so picky.") If, instead, we view these as opportunities to drive improvement – research ethics committees, for instance, are not antiresearch, but pro-human subjects, even if some members rather too much enjoy their power and authority – then we will have taken the correct approach. In any case, one-size-fits-all ethics is inadequate to the task of Big Data.

Bioinformatics and data mining

The flow of information from DNA to RNA to protein to structure involves a great deal of data and information. Humans have as many as 25,000 genes. There are billions of humans. That is a lot of data and information, so much so that one text announces that "Biology, or more generally life sciences, can now be considered information sciences" (Dziuda 2010, 1). Bioinformatics is the use of information technology to study it all. Data mining is a branch of computer science contributing to "knowledge discovery in databases," sometimes called "machine learning." Its algorithms are used to find patterns in large data sets. Definitions of "data mining" variously want these patterns to be "interesting" or "useful."

What is most striking here is the core similarity among running a data mining program, conducting a clinical trial, and sampling a population: At ground, they are all about the identification or even discovery of patterns. All three are of greatest use if they can distinguish signal from noise, filter out (mere) correlations, and identify *causal* patterns or connections. It might very well be that people born on Tuesdays or are Sagittarians have more cancer than people born on Fridays or are Capricorns – and it would be a mistake to make anything of it. But to be able to probe a large genomic, hospital, or linked hospital-genomic data set and derive useful patterns is an exciting opportunity. We can structure a query, the elements of which can range across, well, anything for which we have data:

diagnosis, lab values, single nucleotide polymorphisms, age, occupation, ethnicity, and so on, to derive … well, what? This is, of course, utterly unacceptable in hypothesis-driven science, where hypotheses are tested and sometimes confirmed or falsified (and sometimes wrongly confirmed or falsified). Such a willy-nilly query strategy as rumored here will, on shallow analysis, make it seem that loading a program, framing a question, and hitting the "Enter" key constitute a scientific activity. Empirical science embraced hypothesis testing not for its infallibility but for its ability to filter noise, increase warrant for belief in causal relations, and be replicated or corroborated (or not). To run the same query on the same data set and elicit the same result is no kind of confirmation or corroboration. Moreover, one of the goals of some recent analyses is to identify tools for people with no programming experience (Greene et al. 2014). This goal is not unworthy – it just represents an unsettling change from familiar laboratory practice. Indeed, none of this is to say that data mining in bioinformatics will not deliver the kind of knowledge discovery we want; rather, it is to say that the question whether it will is itself a meta-empirical and methodological one. So our first duty is to study and test the method, and compare it to others. This is no mere stratagem – it is proffered here as an ethical obligation.

Two decades ago an attempt to identify ethical issues in bioinformatics rounded up the usual suspects from "genethics," namely privacy and confidentiality, stigma of population groups and subgroups, data sharing. But it also raised the question of data base accuracy and the problem then of errors in and recanting of linkage analyses; it fretted over quality control (Goodman 1996c). Those suspects are still worthy of interrogation.

Following is a brief list of additional ethical issues at the bioinformatics–data mining seam. Each is under-addressed, at least in the context of bioinformatics, and yet worthy of a sustained analysis elsewhere in the literature.

- *Annotation and curation*: Back in the day, sequences were annotated by hand. Today, if we want tractable or readable data in our datasets,[25] there must be support for "researchers' ability to locate, integrate and access them. In recent years, this challenge has been met by a growing cadre of biologists – 'biocurators' – who manage raw biological data, extract information from published literature, develop structured vocabularies to tag data and make the information available online" (Howe et al. 2008, 48; note omitted; cf. Dolinski et al. 2013). To get this ethically right, we need to do it methodologically right.[26] Relatedly,

- *Interplatform harmonization*: This unintentionally grand label affixes to a simple idea, one central to translational science: Be mindful of the endgames of biomedical research, namely improved patient care and public health. There is nothing wrong with basic research in biology, but if we are going to curate all this data, it would be well if data miners and electronic health record developers, for instance, knew something of each others' trades. Efforts to curate data exclusively for research analysis will miss countless opportunities if they are out of sync with limitations of current electronic health records. If personalized medicine is to keep its many, large, and enthusiastic promises, it will require these translational tools and skills.

- *Be good bioinformaticians*: Here, we want "good" to be parsed as something like "virtuous." In Chapter 4, we proposed a set of "laboratory programmer duties." They are the duties of bioinformaticians, too; in fact these duties are of increased importance to them given the likelihood, eventually, of proximity to patient care. The duties (themselves elaborations of transparency, veracity, and accountability/responsibility) are as follows: write code appropriate to the purpose; annotate, curate, and document carefully; identify provenance; take responsibility as and when appropriate; and attend carefully to version control. If, for instance, we succeed in placing clinically useful genomic information in the electronic health record, the size and complexity of that information will be such as to introduce a new round of challenges (Kho et al. 2013), and quality and quality control may emerge as the greatest ethical challenge of all.

One example of the need to weave these duties throughout the undertaking is available in work not merely on data sets but on promising clinical applications in nanotechnology, specifically nanoproteomics. One assessment points to "(1) immunosensors for inflammatory, pathogenic, and autoimmune markers for infectious and autoimmune diseases, (2) amplified immunoassays for detection of cancer biomarkers, and (3) methods for targeted therapy and automatically adjusted drug delivery such as in experimental stroke and brain injury studies" (Kobeissy et al. 2014). The point at which Big Data analyses lead to uptake in the clinic (Baptista 2014), or where probabilistic analyses guide practice and future research, or where the cost of doing any of this is high and not likely for some time to be widely available, we need to move with caution.

Several reasons support this invocation of "progressive caution" from Chapter 1. Although it is true that science is generally self-correcting, as we have seen earlier, there is sometimes a lot to correct. Besides, although the cost of sequencing a genome has dropped with great rapidity, the cost of clinically useful applications for personalized and targeted medicine has not. Indeed, it is not yet clear what those clinical applications are or will be, our enthusiasm notwithstanding. Yet any attempt at applications will be dear, and someone, or some government, will need to write the check. Contrarily, if our enthusiasm turns out to be justified, then we must, absolutely must, prevent another instance in which an exciting new medical technology actually works – but is available only to those who can pay for it. (For a discussion of the relationship between bioethics and business ethics in bioinformatics, see Goodman and Cava 2008.) The key point here is also that attending to good practice of the kind just earlier itemized also contributes to the cause by helping to reduce at least some need for error correction and management.

Learning health systems, trusted governance, and translational bioscience

This chapter began with an encomium to biomedical research. Whether bent over a laboratory bench, a keyboard, a hospital bed, or a map, scientists and others make observations about the world, or of challenges to and tests of how it works. They learn and share with others. We have also encountered machines that learn. With crowdsourcing and community engagement, we have contemplated what it means for the sources of our data – and targets of our treatments and interventions – to participate in that learning. Now this:

> Progress in computational science, information technology … and biomedical and health research methods have made it possible to foresee the emergence of a learning health system that enables both the seamless and efficient delivery of best care practices and the real-time generation and application of new knowledge. Increases in the complexity and costs of care compel such a system. With rapid advances in approaches to diagnosis (such as molecular diagnostics), therapeutics, genetic insights into individual variation, and

emerging measurement modalities (such as within proteomics and imaging), clinicians and patients must sort through exponentially increasing numbers of factors with each clinical decision. (Institute of Medicine 2011, 1)

This landmark Institute of Medicine report set in motion a suite of efforts to make the most of all the data and information we find and create, and use it for the sake of patients and populations. The anthropomorphization of health systems as "learning systems" captures intuitions of the sort we have been entertaining throughout the present project – fundamentally, the idea that we have an obligation to do a better job using, applying, and evaluating Big Data for improved health. Remember, we are collecting it anyway; the challenge is how to use and reuse it in the best and most appropriate way. It is also a kind of injunction to be mindful of consequent duties, even as we relish the gadgets, tools, and intelligent machines that make it all possible.

At the center of the Institute of Medicine report is its ethical core, a suite of statements about the importance of trust. For instance, under the title "Demonstrating Value to Secure Trust," Ted Shortliffe writes, "We need to understand that the public's support for [electronic health records] depends on their sense that their care is improved or their life is simplified when their provider uses the technology. The public needs to believe that all prudent measures are being taken to ensure that their personal data are protected from loss or inappropriate access" (Shortliffe 2011, 151; cf. Foster 2011; Malin 2011; McGraw 2011). We have already identified and repeatedly explained the essential role of trust in the development and use of health information technology.

More is needed, much more, and, indeed, this is what motivates and justifies the analysis of other ethical issues, as in this book. Other than as noted above, the Institute of Medicine report neither addresses those issues nor does it offer an assessment of how ethics should inform a learning health care system. That task is taken up elsewhere, in a thoughtful analysis of how such a system warrants "a departure from traditional research ethics and clinical ethics" (Faden et al. 2013) with an ethical framework that identifies seven obligations: respect the rights and dignity of patients, respect clinician judgments, provide optimal clinical care to each patient, avoid imposing nonclinical risks and burdens on patients, address health inequalities, conduct continuous learning activities that improve the quality of clinical care and health care systems, and contribute to the common purpose of improving the quality and value of clinical care and health care systems.

At least as important for our purposes, Nancy Kass, Ruth Faden, and colleagues lend important support to the position argued here, namely, that the "received view" that clinical practice and research are distinct is no longer adequate and likely even mistaken: "Requiring only what is classified as research to undergo the burdens and costs of extensive oversight ... creates the situation that we are now in: the policy creates disincentives to rigorous learning, thereby increasing the likelihood that interventions will continue to be introduced into clinical practice and health care systems in the absence of scientific efforts to evaluate their effects" (Kass et al. 2013, S12; citing Baily 2008).

One way to think about the very large next steps required here is to consider work on what have come to be called "trusted governance systems." The problem before us is shaped by the following considerations:

- There are large amounts of data from electronic health records.
- There are increasingly large amounts of data from genomics, some of it in those records, some not.

- We envision a future of digital biobanks, dynamically linked to electronic health records.
- We want to protect all this data and associated transactions from inappropriate uses and users.
- We want as much permission as possible to analyze the data.
- We must foster and sustain public trust in the system.

Trusted governance systems seem to provide the best approach (cf. Platt and Kardia 2015; Williams et al. 2015). One of the core ideas underlying trusted governance is that consent to data use is not well captured with current and standard consent forms, paper or electronic. (Indeed, the current consent process has become so formulaic, sclerosed, and shaped more by legal liability concerns than the need to impart useful information about risks, benefits, and alternatives. It is a wonder there is not greater demand to come up with something different.) Would it not be better to build a publicly familiar and accountable system that obtains as much consent for as much data research as possible at the beginning of a patient's relationship with a health care system, updating as needed or appropriate? Indeed, how fine-grained does consent today need to be for research tomorrow, especially given that the research will be on information, most or all of it de-identified, and therefore of very low risk. Put in the opposite direction: Why not make it easy for ordinary people to contribute to learning health care systems if it is correct to infer that they both want to and have a duty to do so?[27]

There remain many challenges. One is the problem of de- and re-identification of data and information. Data can be stripped of more or less all "unique identifiers" (name, address, and so on). As more information remains there are more privacy concerns, but the less such information that remains, the less use is the data or biological sample. Robust de-identification might be accompanied by assignment of a code number to allow for tracking over time, or so-called "pseudonymization." In all cases, is seems possible that clever (and sometimes not-so-clever) hackers could re-identify any sample or individual-specific data cluster. Efforts to argue that because of this small risk, the collection and analysis of data cannot be permitted, are misguided. The correct response is that better security and control can reduce such already-small risks – and, as previously suggested, the job of applied ethics in these cases is not to say "no," but, rather, "here's how."

This is a period of intense and fertile research on the development of nimble query tools,[28] policies, and frameworks to manage consent, privacy, and other challenges, while producing as much research benefit as possible. For instance, some trusted governance systems include an office or unit, sometimes called the "trusted broker." This unit can provide guidance about privacy and consent, but, most especially, can be of service in the management of "incidental findings" or "unexpected health findings," that is, information about individuals that might be clinically important but which discovery was unexpected. This is closely related to challenges posed by "return of study results." For instance, when the multi-institutional, National Institutes of Health-funded "electronic Medical Records and Genomics" network, or eMERGE, was established in 2007 to "further genomic discovery using biorepositories linked to the electronic health record," it was clear that the project would generate information that would be of use to individual patients (Kullo et al. 2014). The problem of incidental findings is well known in the genetics literature (Ells and Thombs 2014; Wolf 2013), and follows from encountering information that bears non-trivially on individuals – who might or might not want to hear it (sometimes depending whether a treatment or cure for what is found is available) or who have affected relatives where informing the relatives violates the source's confidentiality.[29] These questions, then, whether and when to communicate these findings – perhaps as part of complying with a "duty to warn" – can be quite difficult and will resist any attempt to specify in advance how to manage all of them. Appropriately constituted, a trusted broker unit can provide effective ethical advice regarding communication of incidental findings, help determine the nature of any duty to warn, guide decision makers in assessing whether the scope of an initial consent applies at a later time, and, generally, in making decisions in cases when it is not clear whether or how human-subject protection or privacy laws apply. Providing such services as part of a trusted governance system might come to constitute one of applied ethics' greatest contributions to the growth of biomedical knowledge.

Moreover, the challenge of incidental findings emerged alongside our burgeoning understanding of the difficulties raised by genome research and clinical practice. Those domains alone are rich sources of such challenges. When it comes to fully tractable electronic health record data and information, we haven't seen anything yet.

In the United States, the Clinical and Translational Science Award program commenced in 2006 under the National Center for Advancing Translational Sciences with the goal of improving the bioscience community's ability to link basic research to clinical practice in a bidirectional effort to "catalyze the generation of innovative methods and technologies that will enhance the development, testing and implementation of diagnostics and therapeutics across a wide range of human diseases and conditions."[30] Many of the grantees under this program are, a decade later, seeking ways to develop effective trusted governance systems, these efforts being inspired and guided by the recognition that the development of powerful new technologies in genomics and information technology is an equally powerful generator of ethical challenges.

Innovative and practical ways to address these challenges are essential to keeping the promises made to so many people, ordinary people, who shared their information and, often, quite literally, their blood in hopes of improved health care and a better health care system. Technology and its tools are seductive, treatment gratifying, and discovery exciting. Although the ethical obligations that emerge at the intersection of information technology and bioscience are large, they can be met. We must, however, be on guard against becoming so enthralled by our fantastic new tools that we forget we were supposed to be building something useful, something to improve the health of individuals and of populations.

Notes

1.   Thus: The uncontroversial foundation of consent for clinical practice *and* biomedical research has three components: adequate information (about risks, potential benefits, alternatives), voluntariness (or being able to make a free, uninduced and uncoerced decision), and capacity (or the ability, more or less, to understand and appreciate the information presented and the potential consequences of the decision). Each of these three components is the source of many contributions to the bioethics, medical, and nursing literatures. Because "adequate information" is one of the three components, it renders the phrase "informed consent" less than adequate. One might, for instance, be well informed but under great pressure to give or refuse permission for treatment or research. For this reason, there is growing acceptance of the phrase "valid consent" to describe the process. What made Nazi experiments wrong was the lack of voluntariness. What made the "Tuskegee Study of Untreated Syphilis in the Negro Male" wrong was the absence of adequate information and perhaps of voluntariness. Some experiments in behavioral health have been flawed because of the participants' lack of capacity.

2. That biomedical research is also big business should not be overlooked. In Europe, industry sponsors nearly twice that of governments ($53.6 billion versus $28.1 billion); in the United States, industry spends $70.4 billion versus $48.9 billion in public support (Chakma et al. 2014).

3. Goodman continues:

   Data sharing … collecting and archiving … analysis and reporting … publishing … It seems that the good Dr. Beddoes was calling for a comprehensive system of medical information management. Moreover, he was calling for such a system because he believed, with good warrant, that the medical science of his day was shortchanging – was harming – patients, and that it could be better. Information becomes evidence when it applies to, bears on or constitutes a reason for (dis)believing the truth of a proposition. If we are talking about propositions related to life, death, pain, disability and so forth, then it is just a few short steps until we identify a *duty* to collect and share information that bears on those propositions.

4. Title 45 ("Public Welfare") Code of Federal Regulations, Part 46 ("Protection of Human Subjects") (45 CFR 46.102(d)), 2009 edition, available at www.hhs.gov/ohrp/humansubjects/guidance/45cfr46.html.

5. There is a project in the works to automate (cancer) research itself: "Big Mechanism" has the goal of "reading" and analyzing research papers and generating hypotheses (You 2015).

6. See also Bhatt (2010) and Collier (2009) for reviews of the history of clinical trials. It is suggested that the first trial-like effort is described in the Bible's Book of Daniel, where King Nebuchadnezzar compares the diets of meat eaters and vegetable eaters. After ten days, the vegetarians seemed better off.

7. "There is nothing remarkable in being right in the great majority of cases in the same district, provided the physician knows the signs and can draw the correct conclusions from them" (Hippocrates 1983, cited by Goodman 2003).

8. Personal communication.

9. resilienceproject.me/.

10. It would be a mistake not to mention in passing the debate, if it be that, about the ethical and regulatory differences between surveillance and research. Because surveillance, as by epidemiologists, is not governed by human-subject protection and privacy rules, but research is, the distinction has practical implications. One could argue that absent a very nuanced analysis (as by Hodge and Gostin 2004), it is a distinction without a difference. If the same individuals study the same populations and publish the same results, it is not clear why regulators – and, more importantly, citizens – should care. This is an interesting conceptual question, but it need not detain us.

11. "Ethical Principles and Guidelines for the Protection of Human Subjects of Research," available at www.hhs. gov/ohrp/humansubjects/guidance/belmont.html.

12. From the "Trials of War Criminals before the Nuremberg Military Tribunals under Control Council Law No. 10," Vol. 2, 181–182. Washington, DC: US Government Printing Office, 1949, available at history.nih.gov/ research/downloads/nuremberg.pdf.

13. The report lists two other "basic ethical principles," i.e., "beneficence" and "justice." The report's philosophical foundations lie in the work of the philosopher W.D. Ross, whose "prima facie duties" include several adapted by Tom Beauchamp and Jim Childress, whose modern classic, *Principles of Biomedical Ethics* (2012), elaborates the principles of respect for autonomy, beneficence, nonmaleficence, and justice. Beauchamp wrote much of the Belmont Report.
    It should be pointed out that while *Principles* has probably done more than any other work to introduce health care professionals to bioethics (I once heard a leading health professional exclaim, "How can you do ethics without the principles?!"), they are not universally accepted as the only "way to do bioethics," and, indeed, there are several other approaches with good reasons to be endorsed; they include a common morality and rules approach, casuistry, virtue ethics, and care ethics (or the ethics of care). Suffice it to say that when anyone announces, as if it were settled and received knowledge, that "there are four principles of bioethics and they are these …," she or he is likely mistaken.

14. Notes omitted. The last such, regarding the question why data were not already being used for research, cites Stanley and Meslin (2007).

15. See Barocas and Nissenbaum (2014) for a nuanced and apparently contrary view.

16. The phrase "latent consent" appears to originate in a study of "active" and "passive" methods for obtaining parental permission for children to participate in school activities (Ellickson and Hawes-Dawson 1989).

17. The "Sentinel Initiative aims to develop and implement a proactive system that will complement existing systems that the Agency has in place to track reports of adverse events linked to the use of its regulated products" (www.fda.gov/Safety/FDAsSentinelInitiative/default.htm). "Mini-Sentinel uses pre-existing electronic healthcare data from multiple sources" as a pilot project in support of the Sentinel Initiative (www.mini-sentinel.org/).

18. esphealth.org/ESPnet/images/overview.html.

19. My views on this issue have been shaped in important ways by conversations with Lisa M. Lee. Any misunderstandings and misapplications are mine.

20. Facebook.com. "Information we receive and how it is used," www.facebook.com/about/privacy/your-info.

21. Similarly, the historical origins of advance practice nurses, physicians, surgeons, physician assistants, registered nurses, nursing assistants, and specialists in all of the above are neither scientifically privileged nor, in many instances, particularly efficient. The social, pedagogic, political, and economic forces that generated this menagerie of health professionals are likely contingent; on another planet, they might very well do it all differently, to no ill effect, if not better.

22. It is worth an aside here to inquire why – not to advocate that – the vast health dataverse as fantasized might not be made available to everyone? Imagine this vast super-repository's Web site, query engine, intuitive interface, and helpful guidelines for learning about the health of communities at the framing of a question and the push of a button? Of course, it will be designed to be impossible to identify individuals. A key feature of the site will be a dynamic list of bona fide and peer-reviewed scientific reports that used the repository, accompanied by lay summaries of the research and its current or expected utility, constantly revised and updated. Imagine citizen scientists trying and sharing useful queries, these being vetted and added to the site according as they are useful.

23. www.pcori.org/content/what-we-do.

24. The report identifies four "Ethical principles for data initiatives" and holds that "The use of data in biomedical research and health care should be in accordance with a publicly statable set of morally reasonable expectations and subject to appropriate governance." The principles (with original emphasis, given here in italics):

   • *The set of expectations about how data will be used in a data initiative should be grounded in the principle of respect for persons.* This includes recognition of a person's profound moral interest in controlling others' access to and disclosure of information relating to them held in circumstances they regard as confidential.

   • *The set of expectations about how data will be used in a data initiative should be determined with regard to established human rights.* This will include limitations on the power of states and others to interfere with the privacy of individual citizens in the public interest (including to protect the interests of others).

   • *The set of expectations about how data will be used (or re-used) in a data initiative, and the appropriate measures and procedures for ensuring that those expectations are met, should be determined with the participation of people with morally relevant interests.* This participation should involve giving and receiving public account of the reasons for establishing, conducting and participating in the initiative in a form that is accepted as reasonable by all. Where it is not feasible to engage all those with relevant interests– which will often be the case in practice – the full range of values and interests should be fairly represented.

   • *A data initiative should be subject to effective systems of governance and accountability that are themselves morally justified.* This should include both structures of accountability that invoke legitimate judicial and political authority, and social accountability arising from engagement of people in a society. Maintaining effective accountability must include effective measures for communicating expectations and failures of governance, execution and control to people affected and to the society more widely. (Nuffield Council on Bioethics 2015, 94–95; original emphasis)

25. Note the useful distinction between "machine readable" and "machine tractable" originating in natural language processing (Wilks et al. 1990). To be machine readable is merely to have a searchable file like a dictionary; to be machine tractable is more akin to a database one could use to identify synonyms, find citation information, or learn details about etymology. Cf. Goodman (2003, 90, n. 10).

26. Further:

How information is presented in the literature greatly affects how fast biocurators can identify and curate it. Papers still often report newly cloned genes without providing GenBank IDs or the species from which the genes were cloned. The entities discussed in a paper, including species, genes, proteins, genotypes and phenotypes must be unambiguously identified during curation. For example, using the HUGO Gene Nomenclature Committee resource (www.genenames.org), we find that the human gene CDKN2A has ten literature based synonyms. One of those, p14, is also a synonym for five other genes: CDK2AP2, CTNNBL1, RPP14, S100A9 and SUB1. To confirm the identity of the gene described, curators make inferences from synonyms, sequences, biological context and bibliographic citations. This time-consuming and error-prone step could be eliminated by compliance with data reporting standards. (Howe et al. 2008; notes omitted)

27. Here is how my colleague Robin N. Fiore put it in an internal document developed at the University of Miami's Clinical and Translational Science Institute:

Trusted Governance is the complete set of arrangements to be put in place in order to provide 360-degree stewardship of data entrusted to the research enterprise and to assure the public who are the targets of our recruitment efforts that they can confidently "consent" to unknown future research because they can trust the way [the institution] will handle their data and their privacy. That is, they can consent now … without knowing the exact details of future research. That makes it possible to do longitudinal studies that would otherwise require expensive re-contact and re-consent efforts without the need for a waiver from the IRB, the conditions of such waiver being very restricted.

28. For instance "URIDE," developed by a team at the Center for Computational Science led by Nick Tsinoremas, also from my institution: miamictsi.org/researchers/research-tools/uride.

29. The philosopher Bernie Gert called this "the problem of too much information." This problem is made more interesting according as the information is more or less about a malady or a trait, as discussed with insight by Chuck Culver, and against a background of alleged inadequacies of well-known approaches to bioethics, described by Dan Clouser (cf. note 11). These three are among the coauthors of a useful volume (Gert et al. 1996). Clouser died in 2000, Gert in 2011, and Culver in 2015. With that last death passed a team that made incomparable contributions to the bioethics literature for more than three decades.

30. www.ctsacentral.org/about-us/ncats.

Appendix A AMIA's Code of Professional and Ethical Conduct

Reprinted with permission of Oxford University Press(Goodman et al. 2013).

Introduction

AMIA, as other professional societies, has a long-standing interest in promoting a strong ethical framework for its membership. This white paper presents the latest AMIA Code of Professional and Ethical Conduct. It was approved in November of 2011 by the AMIA Board of Directors. This document constitutes a revision of, and update to, the first code, approved and published in *J Am Med Inform Assoc* in 2007.[1] In an effort to keep pace with the field's vitality, the code presented here is intended to be a dynamic document, and will continue to evolve as AMIA and the field itself evolve. AMIA will publish on its web site this version of the code as part of a process that seeks ongoing response from, and involvement by, AMIA members.

The code is meant to be practical and easily understood, so it is compact and uses general language. Unlike the ethics codes of some professional societies, the AMIA code is not intended to be prescriptive or legislative; it is aspirational, and as such, provides the broad strokes of a set of important ethical principles especially pertinent to the field of biomedical and health informatics. The code is organized around the common roles of AMIA members and the constituents they serve – including patients, students, and others – and with whom they interact. The AMIA Board and the AMIA Ethics Committee encourage members to offer suggestions for improvements and other changes. In this way, the code will continue to progress and best serve AMIA and the larger informatics community.

Codes of ethics for professionals present special challenges in conception and execution. The goal of this code is to lay out the core values of this profession in a way that inspires AMIA members to acknowledge and embrace these values. While the crafting of the code involved many hours of debate about content and scope, the intent is to produce a document which itself does not engender controversy.

The code's authors are aware that all professionals will, from time to time, find themselves in situations shaped by what has been called "dual agency" or "multiple agency." In these circumstances, a professional encounters conflicting duties or loyalties. An informatics professional may have conflicting duties to patients, to colleagues, to society, and to an employer. Few, if any, codes of ethics are nimble enough to provide guidance in such situations. AMIA members have an Ethics Committee which can provide guidance in some circumstances.

AMIA members are professionally diverse,[2] and include those who are, or are in training to be, nurses, physicians, computer scientists, and others. In many cases, these professions have ethics codes.[3–10] The International Medical Informatics Association, an international federation for which AMIA serves as the US representative organization, also has a "Code of Ethics for Health Information Professionals."[11]

This document does not address – but explicitly incorporates – issues covered by other documents and laws bearing on ethics and professional conduct:

- AMIA's "Conflict of Interest Policy,"[12] which governs the organization's employees and leaders as regards some of their financial and other interactions with outside entities.
- The International Committee of Medical Journal Editors' "Uniform Requirements for Manuscripts Submitted to Biomedical Journals."[13] This document is widely accepted as identifying standards for publication and authorship, and is paralleled by the "editorial policies" for the publisher of *J Am Med Inform Assoc*, the BMJ Group.[14]
- Privacy laws. Several sections herein address patient privacy or the rights of patients to view, and control access to, their health information, and these are intended to parallel and make explicit duties under the law. In the USA, for instance, the Privacy Rule under the Health Insurance Portability and Accountability Act,[15] and as amended, lays out many duties for those who are entrusted with health information. Many other countries have similar laws to protect patient data. Informatics professionals are expected to be familiar with and follow the laws governing their practice.

Members of the Ethics Committee are unanimous in the view that those who work in informatics – much as in other health professions – are duty-bound to embrace a patient-centered approach to their work, even if that work does not involve direct patient care or human subjects research. As elsewhere in the health professions, vulnerable populations or those with special needs may be entitled to additional considerations.

The importance of professionalism and ethics has been recognized for millennia by health professionals and organizations, now including information technology professionals. This code of ethics makes clear AMIA's commitment.

Principles of professional and ethical conduct for AMIA members

As a member of AMIA, I acknowledge my professional duty to uphold the following principles of, and guidelines for, ethical conduct.

I. Key ethical guidelines regarding patients, guardians and their authorized representatives (called here collectively "patients").

- A. Given that patients have the right to know about the existence and use of electronic records containing their personal healthcare information, AMIA members involved in patient care should:

  - 1. Not mislead patients about the collection, use, or communication of their healthcare information;
  - 2. Enable and – as appropriate, within reason and the scope of their position and in accord with independent ethical and legal standards – facilitate patients' rights to access, review, and correct their electronic healthcare information. Further, they should:

- B. Advocate and work as appropriate to ensure that health and biomedical information is acquired, stored, analyzed and communicated in a safe, reliable, secure and confidential manner, and that such information management is consistent with applicable laws, local policies, and accepted informatics processing standards.

- C. Never knowingly disclose biomedical data in violation of legal requirements or accepted local confidentiality practices, or in ways that are inconsistent with the explanation of data disclosure and use previously given to the patient. AMIA members should understand that inappropriate disclosure of biomedical information can cause harm, and so should work to prevent such disclosures. Likewise, even if an action does not involve disclosure, one should not use patient data in ways inconsistent with the stated purposes, goals, or intentions of the organization responsible for these data – except as appropriate for approved research, public health or reporting as required under the law.

II. Key ethical guidelines regarding colleagues. AMIA members should:

- A. Endeavor, as appropriate, to support and foster colleagues' and/or team-members' work in a timely, respectful, and conscientious way to support their roles in healthcare and/or research and education;
- B. Advise colleagues and others, as appropriate, about actual or potential information or systems issues (including system flaws, bugs, etc) that affect patient safety or could hinder colleagues' ability to discharge responsibilities to

patients, other colleagues, involved institutions, or other stakeholders;

- C. If a leader:
  - . 1. Be familiar with these guidelines and their applicability to your practice, unit or organization;
  - . 2. Communicate as appropriate about these ethical guidelines to those you lead;
  - . 3. Strive to promote familiarity with, and use of, these ethical guidelines.

III. Key ethical guidelines regarding institutions, employers, business partners and clients (called here collectively "employers"). AMIA members should:

- A. Understand their duties and obligations to current and former employers and fulfill them to the best of their abilities within the bounds of ethical and legal norms.
- B. Understand and appreciate that employers have legal and ethical rights and obligations, including those related to intellectual property. Understand and respect the obligations of their employers, and comply with local policies and procedures to the extent that they do not violate ethical and legal norms.
- C. Inform the employer and act in accordance with ethico-legal mandates and patient rights when employer actions, policies or procedures would violate ethical or legal obligations or agreements made with patients. AMIA's Ethics Committee might be a resource in such cases.

IV. Key ethical guidelines regarding society and regarding research. AMIA members involved in research should:

- A. Be mindful and respectful of the social or public-health implications of their work, ensuring that the greatest good for society is balanced by ethical obligations to individual patients. Seek the advice of institutional ethics committees, AMIA's Ethics Committee or appropriate institutional review boards, as necessary.
- B. Strive as appropriate in the context of one's position to foster the generation of knowledge and biomedical advances through appropriate support for ethical and institutionally approved research efforts.
- C. Know and abide by the applicable governmental regulations and local policies that define ethical research in their professional environment.

V. General professional and ethical guidelines. AMIA members should:

- A. Maintain competence as informatics professionals;

  - . 1. Recognize technical and ethical limitations and seek consultation when needed;
  - . 2. Obtain applicable continuing education;
  - . 3. Contribute to the education and mentoring of students and others, as appropriate for job function.

- B. Strive to encourage the adoption of informatics approaches supported by adequate evidence to improve health and healthcare; and to encourage and support efforts to improve the amount and quality of such evidence.
- C. Be mindful that their work and actions reflect on the profession and on AMIA.

Conclusion

As a matter of personal and professional integrity, adherence to the principles laid out here is expected of all who have the privilege of serving in the field of biomedical and health informatics. While the cornerstone values of professional integrity do not vary among the professions, those whose skills allow them to contribute in one way or another to the health of individuals and populations may be said to have additional responsibilities, and perhaps higher duties.

Acknowledgments

The authors and the AMIA Ethics Committee would like to thank the AMIA Board of Directors for its continuing interest in refining and publishing these guidelines. Kristin Schelin, AMIA's Director of Operations and Programs, provided invaluable support to the Ethics Committee in its work. Comments on the first version of the code were provided by Dan Stein and Kristina Thomas. Members of the AMIA Ethics Committee who contributed to the first version of the code in 2007 include Mureen Allen, MSBS, MS, MA, Joseph Catapano, MD, Oscar Gyde, MD, Carol Hope, PharmD, and Helga Rippen, MD, PhD, MPH. Also, Jane Brokel, PhD, RN, and Betty Chang, DNSc, RN, were authors of the 2007 version and are not otherwise listed here. This version of the code also owes much to members of AMIA's Ethical, Legal and Social Issues (ELSI) Working Group, chaired during the code revision process by Bonnie Kaplan, PhD.

References

1. Hurdle, J.F., Adams, S., Brokel, J., et al. White paper: a code of professional ethical conduct for the American Medical Informatics Association: an AMIA Board of Directors approved white paper. *J Am Med Inform Assoc* 2007;**14**:391–3.

2. Hersh, W. Viewpoint paper: who are the informaticians? What we know and should know. *J Am Med Inform Assoc* 2006;**13**:166–70.

3. American Nurses Association, Code of Ethics for Nurses. 2001. www.nursing world.org/MainMenuCategories/Ethics Standards/CodeofEthicsforNurses.aspx.

4. American College of Physicians, Ethics Manual. 2005. www.acponline.org/run ning_practice/ethics/manual/.

5. American Health Information Management Association, American Health Information Management Association Code of Ethics. 2004; On-line version of the AHIMA Code of Ethics. http://library.ahima.org/xpedio/groups/ public/documents/ahima/bok1_024277. hcsp?dDocName=bok1_024277.

6. Association of Computing Machinery, ACM Code of Ethics and Professional Conduct. 1992. www.acm.org/constitu tion/code.html.

7. Healthcare Information and Management Systems Society, Code of Ethics. 2002. http://ethics.iit.edu/indexOfCodes-2.php? key=13_375_1324.

8. Association of Internet Researchers, Ethical decision-making and Internet Research. 2002. http://aoir.org /reports/ethics.pdf.

9. Medical Library Association, Code of Ethics for Health Sciences Librarianship. 2010. www.mlanet.org /about/ethics.html.

10. Illinois Institute of Technology, Codes of Ethics Online. 2011. http://ethics.iit.edu/ codes/codes_index.html.

11. International Medical Informatics Association, IMIA Code of Ethics for Health Information Professionals. 2002; On-line version of the IMIA Code of Ethics. www.imia-medinfo.org/new2/ node/39.

12. AMIA, Conflict of Interest Policy. 2011. www.amia.org/about-amia/bylaws-and-policies/conflict-interest-policy.

13. International Committee of Medical Journal Editors, Uniform requirements for manuscripts submitted to biomedical journals: writing and editing for biomedical publications. 2010. www.icmje.org.

14. BMJ Group, Editorial Policies. 2011. http://group.bmj.com/products /journals/instructions-for-authors/ editorial-policies/.

15. Health Insurance Portability and Accountability Act of 1996 (Public Law 104–191). http://aspe.hhs.gov/admnsimp/ pl104191.htm .

Appendix B The IMIA Code of Ethics for Health Information Professionals

Reprinted with permission of the International Medical Informatics Association (IMIA).

Preamble

Codes of professional ethics serve several purposes:

1. to provide ethical guidance for the professionals themselves,
2. to furnish a set of principles against which the conduct of the professionals may be measured, and
3. to provide the public with a clear statement of the ethical considerations that should shape the behaviour of the professionals themselves.

A Code of Ethics for Health Informatics Professionals (HIPs) should therefore be clear, unambiguous, and easily applied in practice. Moreover, since the field of informatics is in a state of constant flux, it should be flexible so as to accommodate ongoing changes without sacrificing the applicability of its basic principles. It is therefore inappropriate for a Code of Ethics for HIPs to deal with the specifics of every possible situation that might arise. That would make the Code too unwieldy, too rigid, and too dependent on the current state of informatics. Instead, such a Code should focus on the ethical position of the Health Informatics specialist as a professional, and on the relationships between HIPs and the various parties with whom they interact in a professional capacity. These various parties include (but are not limited to) patients, health care professionals, administrative personnel, health care institutions as well as insurance companies and governmental agencies, etc.

The reason for constructing a code of ethics for HIPs instead of merely adopting one of the codes that have been promulgated by the various general associations of informatics professionals is that HIPs play a unique role in the planning and delivery of health care: a role that is distinct from the role of other informatics professionals who work in different settings.

Part of this uniqueness is centred in the special relationship between the electronic health record (EHR) and the subject of that record. The EHR not only reveals much about the patient that is private and should be kept confidential but, more importantly, it functions as the basis of decisions that have a profound impact on the welfare of the patient. The patient is in a vulnerable position, and any decision regarding the patient and the EHR must acknowledge the fundamental necessity of striking an appropriate balance between ethically justified ends and otherwise appropriate means. Further, the data that are contained in the EHR also provide the raw materials for decision-making by health care institutions, governments and other agencies without which a system of health care delivery simply could not function. The HIP, therefore, by facilitating the construction, maintenance, storage, access, use and manipulation of EHRs, plays a role that is distinct from that of other informatics specialists.

At the same time, precisely because of this facilitating role, HIPs are embedded in a web of relationships that are subject to unique ethical constraints. Thus, over and above the ethical constraints that arise from the relationship between the electronic record and the patient, the ethical conduct of HIPs is also subject to considerations that arise out of the HIPs' interactions with Health Care Professionals (HCPs), health care institutions and other agencies. These constraints pull in different directions. It is therefore important that HIPs have some idea of how to resolve these issues in an appropriate fashion. A Code of Ethics for HIPs provides a tool in this regard, and may be of use in effecting a resolution when conflicting roles and constraints collide.

A Code of Ethics for HIPs is also distinct from an account of legally conferred duties and rights. Unquestionably, the law provides the regulatory setting in which HIPs carry out their activities. However, ethical conduct frequently goes beyond what the law requires. The reason is that legal regulations have purely juridical significance and represent, as it were, a minimum standard as envisioned by legislators, juries and judges. However, these standards are formulated on the basis of circumstances as they obtain here and now; they are not anticipatory in nature and therefore can provide little guidance for a rapidly evolving discipline in which new types of situations constantly arise. HIPs who only followed the law, and who only adjusted their conduct to legal precedent, would be ill equipped to deal with situations that were not envisioned by the lawmakers and would be subject to the vagaries of the next judicial process.

On the other hand, a Code of Ethics for HIPs is grounded in fundamental ethical principles as these apply to the types of situations that characterize the activities of the Health Informatics specialist. Consequently such a Code, centring in the very essence of what it is to be an HIP, is independent of the vagaries of the judicial process and, rather than following it, may well guide it; and rather than becoming invalidated by changes in technology or administrative fashion, may well indicate the direction in which these developments should proceed. Therefore, while in many cases the clauses of such a Code will be reflected in corresponding juridical injunctions or administrative provisions, they provide guidance through times of legal or administrative uncertainty and in areas where corresponding laws or administrative provisions do not exist. At a more general level, such a Code may even assist in the resolution of the problems posed by the technological imperative. Not everything that can be done should be done. A Code of Ethics assists in defining the ethical landscape.

The Code of Ethics that follows was developed on the basis of these considerations. It has two parts:

1. *Introduction*
   This part begins with a set of *fundamental ethical principles* that have found general international acceptance. Next is a brief list of *general principles of informatic ethics that* follow from these fundamental ethical principles when these are applied to the electronic gathering, processing, storing, communicating, using, manipulating and accessing of health information in general. These general principles of informatic ethics are high-level principles and provide general guidance.

2. *Rules of Ethical Conduct for HIPs.*
   This part lays out a detailed set of ethical rules of behaviour for HIPs. These rules are developed by applying the general principles of informatic ethics to the types of relationships that characterize the professional lives of HIPs. They are more specific than the general principles of informatic ethics, and offer more particular guidance.

The precise reasoning that shows how the *Principles of Informatic Ethics* follow from the *Fundamental Ethical Principles,* and that indicates how the *Principles of Informatic Ethics* give rise to the more specific *Rules of Ethical Conduct for HIPs* is contained in a separate *Handbook* and may be consulted there for greater clarity.

It should also be noted that the *Code of Ethics* and the accompanying set of *Rules of Ethical Conduct* do not include what might be called "technical" provisions. That is to say, they do not make reference to such things as technical standards of secure data communication, or to provisions that are necessary to ensure a high quality in the handling, collecting, storing, transmitting, manipulating, etc. of health care data. This is deliberate. While the development and implementation of technical standards has ethical dimensions, and while these dimensions are reflected in the *Code* and the *Rules* as ethical duties, the details of such technical standards are not themselves a matter of ethics.

Part I Introduction
A Fundamental Ethical Principles
All social interactions are subject to fundamental ethical principles. HIPs function in a social setting. Consequently, their actions are also subject to these principles. The most important of these principles are:

1. *Principle of Autonomy*
   All persons have a fundamental right to self-determination.
2. *Principle of Equality and Justice*
   All persons are equal as persons and have a right to be treated accordingly.
3. *Principle of Beneficence*
   All persons have a duty to advance the good of others where the nature of this good is in keeping with the fundamental and ethically defensible values of the affected party.

4. *Principle of Non-Maleficence*
   All persons have a duty to prevent harm to other persons insofar as it lies within their power to do so without undue harm to themselves.
5. *Principle of Impossibility*
   All rights and duties hold subject to the condition that it is possible to meet them under the circumstances that obtain.
6. *Principle of Integrity*
   Whoever has an obligation, has a duty to fulfil that obligation to the best of her or his ability.

B General Principles of Informatic Ethics
These fundamental ethical principles, when applied to the types of situations that characterize the informatics setting, give rise to general ethical principles of informatic ethics.

1. *Principle of Information-Privacy and Disposition*
   All persons have a fundamental right to privacy, and hence to control over the collection, storage, access, use, communication, manipulation and disposition of data about themselves.
2. *Principle of Openness*
   The collection, storage, access, use, communication, manipulation and disposition of personal data must be disclosed in an appropriate and timely fashion to the subject of those data.
3. *Principle of Security*
   Data that have been legitimately collected about a person should be protected by all reasonable and appropriate measures against loss, degradation, unauthorized destruction, access, use, manipulation, modification or communication.
4. *Principle of Access*
   The subject of an electronic record has the right of access to that record and the

right to correct the record with respect to its accurateness, completeness and relevance.

5. *Principle of Legitimate Infringement*
   The fundamental right of control over the collection, storage, access, use, manipulation, communication and disposition of personal data is conditioned only by the legitimate, appropriate and relevant data-needs of a free, responsible and democratic society, and by the equal and competing rights of other persons.

6. *Principle of the Least Intrusive Alternative*
   Any infringement of the privacy rights of the individual person, and of the individual's right to control over person-relative data as mandated under *Principle 1*, may only occur in the least intrusive fashion and with a minimum of interference with the rights of the affected person.

7. *Principle of Accountability*
   Any infringement of the privacy rights of the individual person, and of the right to control over person-relative data, must be justified to the affected person in good time and in an appropriate fashion.

These general principles of informatic ethics, when applied to the types of relationships into which HIPs enter in their professional lives, and to the types of situations that they encounter when thus engaged, give rise to more specific ethical duties. The *Rules of Conduct for HIPs* that follow outline the more important of these ethical duties. It should be noted that as with any ethical rules of conduct, the *Rules* cannot do more than provide guidance. The precise way in which the *Rules* apply in a given context, and the precise nature of a particular ethical right or obligation, depends on the specific nature of the relevant situation.

Part II Rules of Ethical Conduct for HIPs

The rules of ethical conduct for HIPs can be broken down into six general rubrics, each of which has various sub-sections. The general rubrics demarcate the different domains of the ethical relationships that obtain between HIPs and specific stakeholders; the sub-sections detail the specifics of these relationships.

A Subject-centred duties

These are duties that derive from the relationship in which HIPs stand to the subjects of the electronic records or to the subjects of the electronic communications that are facilitated by the HIPs through their professional actions.

1. HIPs have a duty to ensure that the potential subjects of electronic records are aware of the existence of systems, programmes or devices whose purpose it is to collect and/or communicate data about them.

2. HIPs have a duty to ensure that appropriate procedures are in place so that:

   a. electronic records are established or communicated only with the voluntary, competent and informed consent of the subjects of those records, and

   b. if an electronic record is established or communicated in contravention of A.2.a, the need to establish or communicate such a record has been demonstrated on independent ethical grounds to the subject of the record, in good time and in an appropriate fashion.

3. HIPs have a duty to ensure that the subject of an electronic record is made aware that

   a. an electronic record has been established about her/him,

b. who has established the record and who continues to maintain it,

c. what is contained in the electronic record,

d. the purpose for which it is established,

e. the individuals, institutions or agencies who have access to it or to whom it (or an identifiable part of it) may be communicated,

f. where the electronic record is maintained,

g. the length of time it will be maintained, and

h. the ultimate nature of its disposition.

4. HIPs have a duty to ensure that the subject of an electronic record is aware of the origin of the data contained in the record.

5. HIPs have a duty to ensure that the subject of an electronic record is aware of any rights that he or she may have with respect to

a. access, use and storage,

b. communication and manipulation,

c. quality and correction, and

d. disposition

of her or his electronic record and of the data contained in it.

6. HIPs have a duty to ensure that

a. electronic records are stored, accessed, used, manipulated or communicated only for legitimate purposes;

b. there are appropriate protocols and mechanisms in place to monitor the storage, accessing, use, manipulation or communication of electronic records, or of the data contained in them, in accordance with section A.6.a;

c. there are appropriating protocols and mechanisms in place to act on

the basis of the information under section **A.6.b** as and when the occasion demands;

d. the existence of these protocols and mechanisms is known to the subjects of electronic records, and

e. there are appropriate means for subjects of electronic records to enquire into and to engage the relevant review protocols and mechanisms.

7. HIPs have a duty to treat the duly empowered representatives of the subjects of electronic records as though they had the same rights concerning the electronic records as the subjects of the record themselves, and that the duly empowered representatives (and, if appropriate, the subjects of the records themselves) are aware of this fact.

8. HIPs have a duty to ensure that all electronic records are treated in a just, fair and equitable fashion.

9. HIPs have a duty to ensure that appropriate measures are in place that may reasonably be expected to safeguard the

a. security,

b. integrity,

c. material quality,

d. usability, and

e. accessibility

of electronic records.

10. HIPs have a duty to ensure, insofar as this lies within their power, that an electronic record or the data contained in it are used only

a. for the stated purposes for which the data were collected, or

b. for purposes that are otherwise ethically defensible.

11. HIPs have a duty to ensure that the subjects of electronic records or

communications are aware of possible breaches of the preceding duties and the reason for them.

B Duties towards HCPs

HCPs who care for patients depend on the technological skills of HIPs in the fulfilment of their patient-centred obligations. Consequently, HIPs have an obligation to assist these HCPs insofar as this is compatible with the HIPs' primary duty towards the subjects of the electronic records. Specifically, this means that

1. HIPs have a duty
   a. to assist duly empowered HCPs who are engaged in patient care in having appropriate, timely and secure access to relevant electronic records (or parts of thereof), and to ensure the usability, integrity, and highest possible technical quality of these records; and
   b. to provide those informatic services that might be necessary for the HCPs to carry out their mandate.
2. HIPs should keep HCPs informed of the status of the informatic services on which the HCPs rely, and immediately advise them of any problems or difficulties that might be associated or that could reasonably be expected to arise in connection with these informatic services.
3. HIPs should advise the HCPs with whom they interact on a professional basis, or for whom they provide professional services, of any circumstances that might prejudice the objectivity of the advice they give or that might impair the nature or quality of the services that they perform for the HCPs.
4. HIPs have a general duty to foster an environment that is conducive to the maintenance of the highest possible

ethical and material standards of data collection, storage, management, communication and use by HCPs within the health care setting.

5. HCPs who are directly involved in the construction of electronic records may have an intellectual property right in certain formal features of these records. Consequently, HIPs have a duty to safeguard
   a. those formal features of the electronic record, or
   b. those formal features of the data collection, retrieval, storage or usage system in which the electronic record is embedded

   in which the HCP has, or may reasonably be expected to have, an intellectual property interest.

C Duties towards institutions/employers

1. HIPs owe their employers and the institutions in which they work a duty of
   a. competence,
   b. diligence,
   c. integrity, and
   d. loyalty.
2. HIPs have a duty to
   a. foster an ethically sensitive security culture in the institutional setting in which they practice their profession,
   b. facilitate the planning and implementation of the best and most appropriate data security measures possible for the institutional setting in which they work,
   c. implement and maintain the highest possible qualitative standards of data collection, storage, retrieval, processing, accessing, communication and utilization in all areas of their professional endeavour.

3. HIPs have a duty to ensure, to the best of their ability, that appropriate structures are in place to evaluate the technical, legal and ethical acceptability of the data-collection, storage, retrieval, processing, accessing, communication, and utilization of data in the settings in which they carry out their work or with which they are affiliated.

4. HIPs have a duty to alert, in good time and in a suitable manner, appropriately placed decision-makers of the security- and quality-status of the data-generating, storing, accessing, handling and communication systems, programmes, devices or procedures of the institution with which they are affiliated or of the employers for whom they provide professional services.

5. HIPs should immediately inform the institutions with which they are affiliated or the employers for whom they provide a professional service of any problems or difficulties that could reasonably be expected to arise in connection with the performance of their contractually stipulated services.

6. HIPs should immediately inform the institutions with which they are affiliated or the employers for whom they provide a professional service of circumstances that might prejudice the objectivity of the advice they give.

7. Except in emergencies, HIPs should only provide services in their areas of competence; however, they should always be honest and forthright about their education, experience or training.

8. HIPs should only use suitable and ethically acquired or developed tools, techniques or devices in the execution of their duties.

9. HIPs have a duty to assist in the development and provision of appropriate informatics-oriented educational services in the institution which they are affiliated or for the employer for whom they work.

D Duties towards society

1. HIPs have a duty to facilitate the appropriate
   a. collection,
   b. storage,
   c. communication,
   d. use, and
   e. manipulation

   of health care data that are necessary for the planning and providing of health care services on a social scale.

2. HIPs have a duty to ensure that
   a. only data that are relevant to legitimate planning needs are collected;
   b. the data that are collected are de-identified or rendered anonymous as much as possible, in keeping with the legitimate aims of the collection;
   c. the linkage of databases can occur only for otherwise legitimate and defensible reasons that do not violate the fundamental rights of the subjects of the records; and
   d. only duly authorised persons have access to the relevant data.

3. HIPs have a duty to educate the public about the various issues associated with the nature, collection, storage and use of electronic health-data and to make society aware of any problems, dangers, implications or limitations that might reasonably be associated with the collection, storage, usage and manipulation of socially relevant health data.

4. HIPs will refuse to participate in or support practices that violate human rights.

5. HIPs will be responsible in setting the fee for their services and in their demands for working conditions, benefits, etc.

E Self-regarding duties
HIPs have a duty to
1. recognize the limits of their competence,
2. consult when necessary or appropriate,
3. maintain competence,
4. take responsibility for all actions performed by them or under their control,
5. avoid conflict of interest,
6. give appropriate credit for work done, and
7. act with honesty, integrity and diligence.

F Duties towards the profession
1. HIPs have a duty always to act in such a fashion as not to bring the profession into disrepute.
2. HIPs have a duty to assist in the development of the highest possible standards of professional competence, to ensure that these standards are publicly known, and to see that they are applied in an impartial and transparent manner.
3. HIPs will refrain from impugning the reputation of colleagues but will report to the appropriate authority any unprofessional conduct by a colleague.
4. HIPs have a duty to assist their colleagues in living up to the highest technical and ethical standards of the profession.
5. HIPs have a duty to promote the understanding, appropriate utilization, and ethical use of health information technologies, and to advance and further the discipline of Health Informatics.

References

Abaidoo, B., Larweh, B.T. 2014. Consumer health informatics: The application of ICT in improving patient-provider partnership for a better health care. *Online Journal of Public Health Informatics* 16;6(2):e188. doi: 10.5210/ojphi.v6i2.4903.

Abelson, R., Creswell, J. 2015. Data breach at anthem may lead to others. *The New York Times*, February 6, available at www.nytimes. com/2015/02/07/business/data-breach-at-anthem-may-lead-to-others.html?_r=0.

AHIMA. 2009. Auditing copy and paste. *Journal of AHIMA* 80(1):26–9.

Al-Awqati, Q. 2006. How to write a case report: lessons from 1600 B.C. *Kidney International* 69(12):2113–4.

Allen, A. 1988. *Uneasy Access: Privacy for Women in a Free Society*. Totowa, NJ: Rowman & Littlefield.

Alpert, S. 1993. Smart cards, smarter policy: medical records, privacy, and health care reform. *Hastings Center Report* 23(6):13–23.

Alpert, S. 1995. Privacy and intelligent highways: finding the right of way. *Santa Clara Computer & High Technology Law Journal* 11(1):97–118.

Alpert, S. 1998. Health care information: access, confidentiality, and good practice. In Goodman, K.W., ed., *Ethics, Computing and Medicine: Informatics and the Transformation of Health Care*. Cambridge: Cambridge University Press, 75–101.

Amber, K.T., Dhiman, G., Goodman, K.W. 2014. Conflict of interest in online point-of-care clinical support websites. *Journal of Medical Ethics* 40(8):578–80.

American Medical Association. 1910 [copyright and publication date uncertain]. *Nostrums and Quackery: articles on the nostrum evil and quackery reprinted from The Journal of the American Medical Association*. Chicago: American Medical Association, available at https://archive.org/details/nostrumsquackery00amerrich.

American Medical Association. 2014. *Improving Care: Priorities to Improve Electronic Health Record Usability*. Chicago: American Medical Association, available at https://download. ama-assn. org/resources/doc/ps2/x-pub/ehr-priorities.pdf.

Anderson, M., Anderson, S.L., eds. 2011. *Machine Ethics*. Cambridge: Cambridge University Press.

Anderson, J.G., Aydin, C.E. 1994. Overview: theoretical perspectives and methodologies for the evaluation of health care information systems. In Anderson, J.G., Aydin, C.E., Jay, S.J., eds., *Evaluating Health Care Information Systems: Methods and Applications*. Thousand Oaks, CA: Sage, 346–54.

Anderson, J.G., Aydin, C.E. 1998. Evaluating medical information systems: social contexts and ethical challenges. In Goodman, K.W., ed., *Ethics, Computing, and Medicine: Informatics and the Transformation of Health Care*. Cambridge: Cambridge University Press, 57–74.

Anderson, J.G., Goodman, K.W. 2002. *Ethics and Informatics: A Case-Study Approach to a Health System in Transition*. New York: Springer.

Angst, C.M. 2009. Protect my privacy or support the common-good? Ethical questions about electronic health information exchanges. *Journal of Business Ethics* 90:169–78.

Asimov, I. 1950. *I, Robot*. Greenwich, CT.: Fawcett Crest.

Atherton, H., Sawmynaden, P., Sheikh, A., Majeed, A., Car, J. 2012. Email for clinical communication between patients/caregivers and healthcare professionals. *Cochrane Database of Systematic Reviews*, November 14, 2011:CD007978, available at http://online library.wiley.com/doi/10.1002/14651858. CD007978.pub2/abstract.

Atreya, R.V., Smith, J.C., McCoy, A.B., Malin, B., Miller, R.A. 2013. Reducing patient re-identification risk for laboratory results within research datasets. *Journal of the American Medical Informatics Association* 20(1):95–101.

Augestad, K.M., Berntsen, G., Lassen, K., Bellika, J.G., Wootton, R., Lindsetmo, R.O., Study

Group of Research Quality in Medical Informatics and Decision Support (SQUID). 2012. Standards for reporting randomized controlled trials in medical informatics: a systematic review of CONSORT adherence in RCTs on clinical decision support. *Journal of the American Medical Informatics Association* **19**(1):13–21.

Baily, M.A. 2008. Harming through protection? *New England Journal of Medicine* **358**(8):768–9.

Baker, L., Wagner, T.H., Singer, S., Bundorf, M. K. 2003. Use of the Internet and e-mail for health care information: results from a national survey. *Journal of the American Medical Association* **289**(18):2400–6.

Baldwin, T.T., Magjuka, R.J., Loher, B.T. 1991. The perils of participation: effects of choice of training on trainee motivation and learning. *Personnel Psychology* **44**(1):51–65.

Baptista, P.V. 2014. Nanodiagnostics: leaving the research lab to enter the clinics? *Diagnosis* **1**(1):305–9.

Barocas, S., Nissenbaum, H. 2014. Big Data's end run around anonymity and consent. In Lane, J., Stodden, V., Bender, S., Nissenbaum, H., eds., *Privacy, Big Data, and the Public Good*. New York: Cambridge University Press, 44–75.

Baron, J. 1998. *Judgment Misguided: Intuition and Error in Public Decision Making*. New York: Oxford University Press.

Bastani, A., Shaqiri, B., Palomba, K., Bananno, D., Anderson, W. 2014. An ED scribe program is able to improve throughput time and patient satisfaction. *American Journal of Emergency Medicine* **32**(5):399–402.

Bates, D.W., Bitton, A. 2010. The future of health information technology in the patient-centered medical home. *Health Affairs* **29**(4):614–21.

Bayer, R., Fairchild, A. 2002. The limits of privacy: surveillance and the control of disease. *Health Care Analysis* **10**:19–35.

Bayer, R., Santelli, J., Klitzman, R. 2015. New challenges for electronic health records: confidentiality and access to sensitive health information about parents and adolescents. *Journal of the American Medical Association* **313**(1):29–30.

Beauchamp, T.L., Childress, J.F. 2012. *Principles of Biomedical Ethics*. 7th edn. Oxford: Oxford University Press.

Beck, F., Richard, J.-B., Nguyen-Thanh, V., Montagni, I., Parizot, I., Renahy, E. 2014. Use of the Internet as a health information resource among French young adults: results from a nationally representative survey. *Journal of Medical Internet Research* **16**(5):e128.

Bellow, S. 1977. *To Jerusalem and Back: A Personal Account*. New York: Avon.

Benitez, K., Malin, B. 2010. Evaluating re-identification risks with respect to the HIPAA privacy rule. *Journal of the American Medical Informatics Association* **17**:169–77.

Beratarrechea, A., Lee, A.G., Willner, J.M., Jahangir, E., Ciapponi, A., Rubinstein, A. 2014. The impact of mobile health interventions on chronic disease outcomes in developing countries: a systematic review. *Telemedicine Journal and E-Health* **20**(1):75–82.

Bernat, J.L. 2013. Ethical and quality pitfalls in electronic health records. *Neurology* **80**(11):1057–61.

Berner, E.S. 2002. Ethical and legal issues in the use of clinical decision support systems. *Journal of Healthcare Information Management* **16**(4):34–7.

Berner, E.S., ed. 2007. *Clinical Decision Support Systems: Theory and Practice*. 2nd edn. New York: Springer.

Berner, E.S. 2014. What can be done to increase the use of diagnostic decision support systems? *Diagnosis* **1**(1):119–23.

Berner, E.S., Maisiak, R.S., Cobbs, C.G., Taunton, O.D. 1999. Effects of a decision support system on physicians' diagnostic performance. *Journal of the American Medical Informatics Association* **6**:420–7.

Berner, E.S., Webster, G.D., Shugerman, A.A., Jackson, J.R., Algina, J., Baker, A.L. 1994. Performance of four computer-based diagnostic systems. *New England Journal of Medicine* **330**:1792–6.

Bhatia, H.L., Patel, N.R., Choma, N.N., Grande, J., Giuse, D.A., Lehmann, C.U. 2015. Code status and resuscitation options in the electronic health record. *Resuscitation* **87**:14–20

Bhatt, A. 2010. Evolution of Clinical Research: A history before and beyond James Lind. *Perspectives in Clinical Research* **1**(1):6–10.

Bilimoria, N.M. 2009. HIPAA Privacy/Security Rules: where we've been and where we are going. Updates from the HITECH Act to dramatically impact HIPAA privacy/security. *Journal of Medical Practice Management* 25(3):149–52.

BMJ. 1998. The hippocratic oath (editorial). *BMJ* 317:1110.

BMJ. 2001. Medical oaths and declarations (editorial). *BMJ* 323:1440.

BMJ. 2009. Surgical training using simulation (editorial). *BMJ* 338:b1001.

Boguski, M.S., Mandl, K.D., Sukhatme, V.P. 2009. Repurposing with a difference. *Science* 324(5933):1394–5.

Bok, S. 1983. *Secrets: On the Ethics of Concealment and Revelation.* New York: Vintage Books/Random House.

Borenstein, J., Pearson, Y. 2012. Robot caregivers: Ethical issues across the human lifespan. In Abney, K., Bekey, G.A., eds., *Robot Ethics: The Ethical and Social Implications of Robots.* Cambridge, MA: MIT Press, 251–65.

Boudreaux, E.D., Waring, M.E., Hayes, R.B., Sadasivam, R.S., Mullen, S., Pagoto, S. 2014. Evaluating and selecting mobile health apps: strategies for healthcare providers and healthcare organizations. *Translational Behavioral Medicine* 4(4):363–71.

Bower, J.L., Christensen, C.M. 1995. Disruptive technologies: catching the wave. *Harvard Business Review* 73(1):43–53.

Boyd, J.E., Adler, E.P., Otilingam, P.G., Peters, T. 2014. Internalized Stigma of Mental Illness (ISMI) scale: a multinational review. *Comprehensive Psychiatry* 55(1):221–31.

Brady, K., Shariff, A. 2013. Virtual medical scribes: making electronic medical records work for you. *Journal of Medical Practice Management* 29(2):133–6.

Bredillet, C.N. 2003. Genesis and role of standards: theoretical foundations and socio-economical model for the construction and use of standards. *International Journal of Project Management* 21(6):463–70.

Brennan, P.F., Downs, S., Casper, G. 2010. Project Health Design: rethinking the power and potential of personal health records. *Journal of Biomedical Informatics* 43(5 Suppl):S3-5.

Brody, B.A. 1989. The ethics of using ICU scoring systems in individual patient management. *Problems in Critical Care* 3:662–70.

Brooks, F.P. 1995. *The Mythical Man-Month: Essays on Software Engineering Anniversary Edition.* Boston: Addison-Wesley.

Brown, J., Ryan, C., Harris, A. 2014. How doctors view and use social media: a national survey. *Journal of Medical Internet Research* 16(12):e267.

Brownstein, J.S., Freifeld, C.C., Madoff, L.C. 2009. Digital disease detection – harnessing the Web for public health surveillance. *New England Journal of Medicine* 360(21):2153–7.

Bryant, A.D., Fletcher, G.S., Payne, T.H. 2014. Drug interaction alert override rates in the Meaningful Use era: no evidence of progress. *Applied Clinical Informatics* 5(3):802–13.

Bulaj, Z.J., Phillips, J.D., Ajioka, R.S., Franklin, M.R., Griffen, L.M., Guinee, D.J., Edwards, C.Q., Kushner, J.P. 2000. Hemochromatosis genes and other factors contributing to the pathogenesis of porphyria cutanea tarda. *Blood* 95:1565–71.

Bundorf, M.K., Wagner, T.H., Singer, S.J., Baker, L.C. 2006. Who searches the internet for health information? *Health Services Research* 41(3 Pt. 1):819–36.

Carrión Señor, I., Fernández-Alemán, J.L., Toval, A. 2012. Are personal health records safe? A review of free web-accessible personal health record privacy policies. *Journal of Medical Internet Research* 14(4):e114.

CBC. 2011. Online health advice sought by more Canadians, available at www.cbc.ca/news/online-health-advice-sought-by-more-canadians-1.982301.

Chakma, J., Sun, G.H., Steinberg, J.D., Sammut, S.M., Jagsi, R. 2014. Asia's ascent – global trends in biomedical R&D expenditures. *New England Journal of Medicine* 370 (1):3–6.

Chalmers, I., Clarke, M. 2004. Commentary: the 1944 patulin trial: the first properly controlled multicentre trial conducted under the aegis of the British Medical Research Council. *International Journal of Epidemiology* 33(2):253–60.

Cho, I., Park, H., Choi, Y.J., Hwang, M.H., Bates, D.W. 2014. Understanding the nature of medication errors in an ICU with a computerized physician order entry system. *PLoS One* 9(12):e114243.

Christensen, C.M. 1997 *The Innovator's Dilemma: When New Technologies Cause Great Firms to Fail.* Boston: Harvard Business School Press.

Clark, P.A., Capuzzi, K., Harrison, J. 2010. Telemedicine: Medical, legal and ethical perspectives. *Medical Science Monitor* **16**(12): RA261–72.

Clendening, L. 1942. *Source Book of Medical History*. New York: Dover.

Cleveringa, F.G., Gorter, K.J., van den Donk, M., van Gijsel, J., Rutten, G.E. 2013. Computerized decision support systems in primary care for type 2 diabetes patients only improve patients' outcomes when combined with feedback on performance and case management: a systematic review. *Diabetes Technology & Therapeutics* **15**(2):180–92.

Cline, R.J.W., Haynes, K.M. 2001. Consumer health information seeking on the Internet: the state of the art. *Health Education Research* **16**(6):671–92.

Cochrane, A.L. 1979. 1931–1971: a critical review, with particular reference to the medical profession. In *Medicines for the year 2000*. London: Office of Health Economics, 1–11.

Coeckelbergh, M. 2010. Health care, capabilities, and AI assistive technologies. *Ethical Theory and Moral Practice* **13**(2):181–90.

Cohen, D. 2013. Devices and desires: industry fights toughening of medical device regulation in Europe. *BMJ* **347**:f6204.

Cohn, J. 2013. The robot will see you now. *The Atlantic*, March, available at www.theatlantic.com/magazine/archive/2013/03/the-robot-will-see-you-now/309216/.

Collier, R. 2009. Legumes, lemons and streptomycin: a short history of the clinical trial. *Canadian Medical Association Journal* **180**(1):23–4.

Collins, G.S., Reitsma, J.B., Altman, D.G., Moons, K.G.M. 2015. Transparent Reporting of a multivariable prediction model for Individual Prognosis Or Diagnosis (TRIPOD): The TRIPOD Statement. *Annals of Internal Medicine* **162**(1)55–63.

Collins, F.S., Tabak, L.A. 2014. Policy: NIH plans to enhance reproducibility. *Nature* **505**:612–3.

Collste, G., ed. 2000. *Ethics in the Age of Information Technology*. Studies in Applied Ethics 7. Linköping: Centre for Applied Ethics.

Cook, R.I. 2012. Dissenting statement: Health IT is a Class III medical device. In Institute of Medicine. *Health IT and Patient Safety: Building Safer Systems for Better Care*. Washington, DC: The National Academies Press, 193–7.

Cook, D.A., Hatala, R., Brydges, R., Zendejas, B., Szostek, J.H., Wang, A.T., Erwin, P.J., Hamstra, S.J. 2011. Technology-enhanced simulation for health professions education: a systematic review and meta-analysis. *Journal of the American Medical Association* **306**(9):978–88.

Coorevits, P., Sundgren, M., Klein, G.O., Bahr, A., Claerhout, B., Daniel, C., Dugas, M., Dupont, D., Schmidt, A., Singleton, P., De Moor, G., Kalra, D. 2013. Electronic health records: new opportunities for clinical research. *Journal of Internal Medicine* **274**(6):547–60.

Cornet, G. 2013. Robot companions and ethics: a pragmatic approach of ethical design. *Journal international de bioéthique* **24**(4):49–58, 179–80.

Council of Europe. 1981. *Convention for the Protection of Individuals with regard to Automatic Processing of Personal Data*. Strasbourg: Council of Europe, available at http://conventions.coe.int/Treaty/en/Treaties/Html/108.htm.

Curtis, L.H., Brown, J., Platt, R. 2014. Four health data networks illustrate the potential for a shared national multipurpose big-data network. *Health Affairs* **33**(7):1178–86

Cushman, R., Froomkin, A.M., Cava, A., Abril, P., Goodman, K.W. 2010. Ethical, legal and social issues for personal health records and applications. *Journal of Biomedical Informatics* **43**(5 Suppl):S51–5.

Datteri, E. 2013. Predicting the long-term effects of human-robot interaction: a reflection on responsibility in medical robotics. *Science & Engineering Ethics* **19**(1):139–60.

Dautenhahn, K. 2007. Socially intelligent robots: dimensions of human-robot interaction. *Philosophical Transactions of the Royal Society of London. Series B: Biological Sciences* **362**(1480):679–704.

David, P.A., Steinmueller, W.E. 1994. Economics of compatibility standards and competition in telecommunication networks. *Information Economics and Policy* **6**(3–4):217–41.

DeAngelis, C.D. 2014. The electronic health record: boon or bust for good patient care? *The Milbank Quarterly* **92**(3):442–45.

de Dombal, F.T. 1987. Ethical considerations concerning computers in medicine in the 1980s. *Journal of Medical Ethics* **13**:179–84.

de Lusignan, S., Mold, F., Sheikh, A., Majeed, A., Wyatt, J.C., Quinn, T., Cavill, M., Gronlund, T.A., Franco, C., Chauhan, U., Blakey, H., Kataria, N., Barker, F., Ellis, B., Koczan, P., Arvanitis, T.N., McCarthy, M., Jones, S., Rafi, I. 2014. Patients' online access to their electronic health records and linked online services: a systematic interpretative review. *BMJ Open* 4(9):e006021.

De Ville, K.A. 1999. Managed care and the ethics of regulation. *Journal of Medicine and Philosophy* 24(5):492–517.

Devine, E.B., Lee, C.J., Overby, C.L., Abernethy, N., McCune, J., Smith, J.W., Tarczy-Hornoch, P. 2014. Usability evaluation of pharmacogenomics clinical decision support aids and clinical knowledge resources in a computerized provider order entry system: a mixed methods approach. *International Journal of Medical Informatics* 83(7):473–83.

Dhiman, G.J., Amber, K.T., Goodman, K.W. 2015. Comparative outcome studies of clinical decision support software: limitations to the practice of evidence-based system acquisition. *Journal of the American Medical Informatics Association*, February 8. pii:ocu033.

Diero, L., Rotich, J.K., Bii, J., Mamlin, B.W., Einterz, R.M., Kalamai, I.Z., Tierney, W.M. 2006. A computer-based medical record system and personal digital assistants to assess and follow patients with respiratory tract infections visiting a rural Kenyan health centre. *BMC Biomedical Informatics and Decision Making* 6:21.

Dolinski, K., Chatr-aryamontri, S., Tyers, M. 2013. Systematic curation of protein and genetic interaction data for computable biology. *BMC Biology* 11:43.

Donaldson, L. 2003. Expert patients usher in a new era of opportunity for the NHS. *BMJ* 326(7402):1279–80.

Downar, J. 2009. Even without our biases, the outlook for prognostication is grim. *Critical Care* 13(4):168.

Duda, R.O., Shortliffe, E.H. 1983. Expert systems research. *Science* 220:261–8.

Duggan, M., Smith, A. 2013. Social Media Update 2013, available at www.pewinternet.org/files/2013/12/PIP_Social-Networking- 2013.pdf.

Dziuda, D.M. 2010. *Data Mining for Genomics and Proteomics: Analyses of Gene and Protein Expression Data*. Hoboken, NJ: John Wiley & Sons.

Eastwood, G.L. 2009. When relatives and friends ask physicians for medical advice: ethical, legal, and practical considerations. *Journal of General Internal Medicine* 24:1333–5.

Eder, J., Gottweis, H., Zatloukal, K. 2012. IT solutions for privacy protection in biobanking. *Public Health Genomics* 15(5):254–62.

Edworthy, J. 2013. Medical audible alarms: a review. *Journal of the American Medical Informatics Association* 20(3):584–9.

Ellickson, P.L., Hawes-Dawson, J. 1989. *An Assessment of Active Versus Passive Consent for Obtaining Parental Consent*. Santa Monica, CA: RAND.

Elliott, J.E. 1978. Marx's "Grundrisse": vision of capitalism's creative destruction. *Journal of Post Keynesian Economics* 1(2):148–169.

Ells, C., Thombs, B.D. 2014. The ethics of how to manage incidental findings. *Canadian Medical Association Journal* 186(9):655–6.

Embi, P.J., Leonard, A.C. 2012. Evaluating alert fatigue over time to EHR-based clinical trial alerts: findings from a randomized controlled study. *Journal of the American Medical Informatics Association* 19:e145–e148.

Encinosa, W.E., Bae, J. 2015. Meaningful Use IT reduces hospital-caused adverse drug events even at challenged hospitals. *Healthcare* 3(1):12–17.

Engelhardt, H.T. 1985. Typologies of disease: Nosologies revisited. In Schaffner, K.F., ed., *Logic of Discovery and Diagnosis in Medicine*. Berkeley: University of California Press, 56–71.

Epstein, R.A. 1992. The path to "The T. J. Hooper": The theory and history of custom in the law of tort. *The Journal of Legal Studies* 21(1):1–38.

Esposito, K., Goodman, K.W. 2009. Genethics 2.0: Phenotypes, genotypes, and the challenge of databases generated by personal genome testing. *The American Journal of Bioethics* 9(6):19–21.

European Science Foundation. 2011. *The European Code of Conduct for Research Integrity*. Strasbourg: European Science Foundation, available at www.esf.org/fileadmin/Public_documents/Publications/Code_Conduct_ResearchIntegrity.pdf.

Evetts, J. 2013. Professionalism: Value and ideology. *Current Sociology* 61(5–6):778–96.

Faden, R.R., Kass, N.E., Goodman, S.N., Pronovost, P., Tunis, S., Beauchamp, T.L.

2013. An ethics framework for a learning health care system: a departure from traditional research ethics and clinical ethics. *Hastings Center Report* **43**(S1): S16–S27.

Farmer, A.D., Bruckner Holt, C.E., Cook, M.J., Hearing, S.D. 2009. Social networking sites: a novel portal for communication. *Postgraduate Medical Journal* 85(1007):455–9.

Farnan, J.M., Snyder Sulmasy, L., Worster, B.K., Chaudhry, H.J., Rhyne, J.A., Arora, V.M., for the American College of Physicians Ethics, Professionalism and Human Rights Committee. 2013. Online Medical Professionalism: Patient and public relationships: Policy statement from the American College of Physicians and the Federation of State Medical Boards. *Annals of Internal Medicine* 158(8):620–7.

Farr, W. 1837. The Provincial medical and surgical association. *British Annals of Medicine, Pharmacy, Vital Statistics and General Science* 1:692–5.

Farra, R., Sheppard, N.F., McCabe, L., Neer, R. M., Anderson, J.M., Santini, J.T., Cima, M.J., Langer, R. 2012. First-in-human testing of a wirelessly controlled drug delivery microchip. *Science Translational Medicine* 4 (122):122ra21.

Federal Aviation Administration. 2011. *Federal Aviation Administration Task Force on Air Carrier Safety and Pilot Training: Report from the Air Carrier Safety and Pilot Training Aviation Rulemaking Committee*. Washington, DC: Federal Aviation Administration.

Feyerabend, P. 1975/1984. *Against Method*. London: Verso.

Flores, K.E., Quinlan, M.B. 2014. Ethnomedicine of menstruation in rural Dominica, West Indies. *Journal of Ethnopharmacology* **153** (3):624–34.

Floridi, L. 2013. *The Ethics of Information*. Oxford: Oxford University Press.

Fortney, J.C., Burgess, J.F., Bosworth, H.B., Booth, B.M., Kaboli, P.J. 2011. A Re-conceptualization of access for 21st century healthcare. *Journal of General Internal Medicine* 26(Suppl 2):639–47.

Foster, I. 2011. Building a secure learning health system. In Institute of Medicine, *Digital Infrastructure for the Learning Health System: The Foundation for Continuous Improvement in Health and Health Care:*

Workshop Series Summary. Washington, DC: The National Academies Press, 161–4.

Fox, S. 2013. What ails America? Dr. Google can tell you. Pew Research Center, December 17, available at www.pewresearch.org/fact-tank/ 2013/12/17/what-ails-america-dr-google-can-tell-you/.

Fox, S., Duggan, M. 2013. Health Online 2013. Pew Research Center, Pew Internet & American Life Project, available at www.pew internet.org/files/old-media/Files/Reports/ PIP_HealthOnline.pdf.

French, R. 2003. *Medicine before Science: The Business of Medicine from the Middle Ages to the Enlightenment*. Cambridge: Cambridge University Press.

Freshwater, D., Fisher, P., Walsh, E. 2013. Revisiting the Panopticon: professional regulation, surveillance and sousveillance. *Nursing Inquiry*, available at http://online library.wiley.com/doi/10.1111/nin.12038/pdf.

Fried, C. 1968. Privacy (a moral analysis). *Yale Law Journal* 77:475–93.

Friedberg, M.W., Chen, P.G., Van Busum, K.E., Aunon, F., Pham, C., Caloyeras, J., Mattke, S., Pitchforth, E., Quigley, D.D., Brook, R.H., Crosson, F.J., Tutty, M. 2013. *Factors Affecting Physician Professional Satisfaction and Their Implications for Patient Care, Health Systems, and Health Policy*. Rand Corporation Report RR-439-AMA, Santa Monica, CA: Rand Corporation., available at www.rand.org/pubs/ research_reports/ RR439.html.

Friedman, C.P. 2009. A "Fundamental Theorem" of biomedical informatics. *Journal of the American Medical Informatics Association* **16**(2):169–70.

Friend, S.H., Schadt, E.E. 2014. Translational genomics. Clues from the resilient. *Science* 344(6187):970–2.

Fukuyama, F. 2006. *America at the Crossroads: Democracy, Power, and the Neoconservative Legacy*. New Haven: Yale University Press.

Funnell, M.M. 2000. Helping patients take charge of their chronic illnesses. *Family Practice Management* 7(3):47–51.

Galbraith, G.L. 2014. Practical and ethical considerations for using social media in community consultation and public disclosure activities. *Academic Emergency Medicine* 21 (10):1151–7.

Garg, A.X., Adhikari, N.J., McDonald, H., Rosas-Arellano, M.P., Devereaux, P.J.,

Beyene, J., Sam, J., Haynes, R.B. 2005. Effects of computerized clinical decision support systems on practitioner performance and patient outcomes: a systematic review. *Journal of the American Medical Association* 293(10):1223–38.

Gauchat, G. 2012. Politicization of science in the public sphere: A study of public trust in the United States, 1974 to 2010. *American Sociological Review* 77(2):167–87.

Gavison, R. 1984. Privacy and the limits of the law. In Schoeman, F.D., ed., *Philosophical Dimensions of Privacy: An Anthology*. Cambridge: Cambridge University Press, 346–402.

Gellert, G.A., Ramirea, R., Webster, S.L. 2014. The rise of the medical scribe industry: implications for the advancement of electronic health records. *Journal of the American Medical Association*, December 15. doi:10.1001/jama.2014.17128. [Epub ahead of print].

Gert, B., Berger, E.M., Cahill, G.F., Clouser, K. D., Culver, C.M., Moeschler, J.B., Singer, G. H.S. 1996. *Morality and the New Genetics*. Portola Valley, CA: Jones and Bartlett.

Gillum, R.F. 2013. From papyrus to the electronic tablet: A brief history of the clinical medical record with lessons for the digital age. *The American Journal of Medicine* 126:853–7.

Gibbs, S. 2014. Elon Musk: artificial intelligence is our biggest existential threat. *The Guardian*, October 27, available at www.theguardian.com/technology/2014/oct/27/elon-musk-artificial-intelligence-ai-biggest-existential-threat.

Glanzberg, M. 2014. Truth. In Zalta, E.N., ed., *The Stanford Encyclopedia of Philosophy* (Fall 2014 edn.), available at plato.stanford.edu/archives/fall2014/entries/truth.

Glasser, D.J., Goodman, K.W., Einspruch, N.G. 2007. Chips, tags and scanners: Ethical challenges for radio frequency identification. *Ethics and Information Technology* 9:101–9.

Goldman, A.H. 1987. Ethical issues in proprietary restrictions on research results. *Science, Technology and Human Values* 1:22–30.

Goldspiel, B.R., Flegel, W.A., DiPatrizio, G., Sissung, T., Adams, S.D., Penzak, S.R., Biesecker, L.G., Fleisher, T.A., Patel, J.J., Herion, D., Figg, W.D., Lertora, J.J., McKeeby, J.W. 2014. Integrating pharmacogenetic information and clinical decision support into the electronic health record.

Journal of the American Medical Informatics Association 21(3):522–8.

Goldstein, M.M. 2010. Health information technology and the idea of informed consent. *Journal of Law, Medicine & Ethics* 38(1):27–35.

Goodman, K.W. 1993. Intellectual property and control. *Academic Medicine* 68(9):S88–S91.

Goodman, K.W. 1996a. Critical care computing: outcomes, confidentiality, and appropriate use. *Critical Care Clinics* 12:109–22.

Goodman, K.W. 1996b. Codes of ethics in occupational and environmental health. *Journal of Occupational and Environmental Medicine* 38:882–3.

Goodman, K.W. 1996c. Ethics, genomics and information retrieval. *Computers in Biology and Medicine* 26:223–9.

Goodman, K.W., ed. 1998a. *Ethics, Computing and Medicine: Informatics and the Transformation of Health Care*, Cambridge: Cambridge University Press.

Goodman, K.W. 1998b. Bioethics and health informatics: an introduction. In Goodman, K.W., ed., *Ethics, Computing and Medicine: Informatics and the Transformation of Health Care*. Cambridge: Cambridge University Press, 1–31.

Goodman, K.W. 1998c. Outcomes, futility, and health policy research. In Goodman, K.W., ed., *Ethics, Computing and Medicine: Informatics and the Transformation of Health Care*. Cambridge: Cambridge University Press, 116–38.

Goodman, K.W. 1999. Health informatics and the hospital ethics committee. *MD Computing* 16(2):17–20.

Goodman, K.W. 2003. *Ethics and Evidence-Based Medicine: Fallibility and Responsibility in Clinical Science*. Cambridge: Cambridge University Press.

Goodman, K.W. 2010. Ethics, information technology and public health: New challenges for the clinician-patient relationship. *Journal of Law, Medicine and Ethics* 38(1):58–63.

Goodman, K.W. 2011. Health information technology and globalization. In Chadwick, R., ten Have, H., Meslin, E.M., eds., *Health Care Ethics: Core and Emerging Issues*. Los Angeles: Sage, 117–25.

Goodman, K.W. 2014. Health analytics and big data. *Lahey Health Journal of Medical Ethics* Spring:9–10.

Goodman, K.W., Cava, A. 2008. Bioethics, business ethics, and science: Bioinformatics and the future of healthcare. *Cambridge Quarterly of Healthcare Ethics* 17(4):361–72.

Goodman, K.W., Adams, S., Berner, E.S., Embi, P.J., Hsiung, R., Hurdle, J., Jones, D.A., Lehmann, C.U., Maulden, S., Petersen, C., Terrazas, E., Winkelstein, P. 2013. AMIA's Code of Professional and Ethical Conduct. *Journal of the American Medical Informatics Association* 20:141–3.

Goodman, K.W., Berner, E.S., Dente, M.A., Kaplan, B., Koppel, R., Rucker, D., Sands, D.Z., Winkelstein, P. 2011. Challenges in ethics, safety, best practices, and oversight regarding HIT vendors, their customers, and patients: a report of an AMIA special task force. *Journal of the American Medical Informatics Association* 18(1):77–81.

Goodman, K.W., Meslin, E.M. 2014. Ethics, information technology and public health: Duties and challenges in computational epidemiology. In Magnuson, J.A., Fu, P.C., eds., *Public Health Informatics and Information Systems*. 2nd edn. London: Springer, 191–209.

Goodman, K.W., Cushman, R., Miller, R.A. 2014. Ethics in biomedical informatics: users, standards, and outcomes. In Shortliffe, E.H., Cimino, J.J., eds., *Biomedical Informatics: Computer Applications in Health Care and Biomedicine*. 4th edn. New York: Springer, 329–54.

Goodman, K.W., Prineas, R.J. 2009. Ethics curricula in epidemiology. In Coughlin, S.S., Beauchamp, T.L., Weed, D.L., eds., *Ethics and Epidemiology*. 2nd edn. Oxford: Oxford University Press, 283–303.

Gostin, L.O., Hodge, J.G. Jr., Valdiserri, R.O. 2001. Informational privacy and the public's health: the Model State Public Health Privacy Act. *American Journal of Public Health* 91(9):1388–92.

Gostin, L.O., Turek-Brezina, J., Powers, M., Kozloff, R., Faden, R., Steinauer, D. 1993. Privacy and security of personal information in a new health care system. *Journal of the American Medical Association* 270:2487–93.

Gotterbarn, D. 2001. Informatics and professional responsibility. *Science and Engineering Ethics* 7(2):221–30.

Gotz, D., Wang, F., Perer, A. 2014. A methodology for interactive mining and visual analysis of clinical event patterns using electronic health record data. *Journal of Biomedical Informatics* 48:148–59.

Graber, M.L., Wachter, R.M., Cassel, C.K. 2012. Bringing diagnosis into the quality and safety equations. *Journal of the American Medical Association* 308(12):1211–12.

Grajales, F.J., Sheps, S., Ho, K., Novak-Lauscher, H., Eysenbach, G. 2014. Social media: a review and tutorial of applications in medicine and health care. *Journal of Medical Internet Research* 16(2):e13.

Grande, D., Mitra, N., Shah, A., Wan, F., Asch, D.A. 2013. Public preferences about secondary uses of electronic health information. *JAMA Internal Medicine* 173(19):1798–806.

Grande, D., Mitra, N., Shah, A., Wan, F., Asch, D.A. 2014. The importance of purpose: moving beyond consent in the societal use of personal health information. *Annals of Internal Medicine* 161(12):855–62.

Green, M.J., Botkin, J.R. 2003. "Genetic exceptionalism" in medicine: clarifying the differences between genetic and nongenetic tests. *Annals of Internal Medicine* 138(7):571–5.

Greene, R., Mo, K.S., eds. 2006. *The Undead and Philosophy: Chicken Soup for the Soulless.* Chicago: Open Court.

Greene, C.S., Tan, J., Ung, M., Moore, J.H., Cheng, C. 2014. Big data bioinformatics. *Journal of Cell Physiology* 229(12):1896–900.

Greenhalgh, T., Keen, J. 2013. England's national programme for IT. *BMJ* 346:f4130.

Greenwald, J.L, Halasyamani, L., Greene, J., LaCivita, C., Stucky, E., Benjamin, B., Reid, W., Griffin, F.A., Vaida, A.J., Williams, M.V. 2010. Making inpatient medication reconciliation patient centered, clinically relevant and implementable: A consensus statement on key principles and necessary first steps. *Journal of Hospital Medicine* 5(8):477–85.

Greenwood, M. 1948. *Medical statistics from Graunt to Farr.* Cambridge: Cambridge University Press.

Gymrek, M., McGuire, A.L., Golan, D., Halperin, E., Erlich, Y. 2013. Identifying personal genomes by surname inference. *Science* 339(6117):321–4.

Hardwig, J. 1991. The role of trust in knowledge. *The Journal of Philosophy* 84(12):693–707.

Harris, B.L. 1990. Becoming deprofessionalized: One aspect of the staff nurse's perspective on computer-mediated nursing care plans. *Advances in Nursing Science* **13**(2):63–74.

Hartmann, F. 1988. *Paracelsus: Life and Prophecies.* Blauvelt, NY: Steinerbooks, Garber Communications.

Hartzband, P., Groopman, J. 2008. Off the record – avoiding the pitfalls of going electronic. *New England Journal of Medicine* **358**:1656–8.

Hayek, F.A. 2007. *The Road to Serfdom: Text and Documents, The Definitive Edition.* Caldwell, B., ed. Chicago: University of Chicago Press.

Häyry, M., Chadwick, R., Árnason, V., Árnason, G. 2007. *The Ethics and Governance of Human Genetic Databases.* Cambridge: Cambridge University Press.

Hébert, P.C., Levin, A.V., Robertson, G. 2001. Bioethics for clinicians: 23. Disclosure of medical error. *Canadian Medical Association Journal* **164**(4):509–13.

Hettrick, S. 2014. It's impossible to conduct research without software, say 7 out of 10 UK researchers. Software Sustainability Institute, available at www.software.ac.uk/blog/2014-12-04-its-impossible-conduct-research-without-software-say-7-out-10-uk-researchers.

Hew, F.C. 2014. Artificial moral agents are infeasible with foresee technologies. *Ethics and Information Technology* **1**:197–206.

Heyman, J. 2010. Health IT and solo practice: A love-hate relationship. *Journal of Law, Medicine & Ethics* **38**(1):14–16.

Hilkevitch, J. 2012. Technology may be eroding pilot skills. *Chicago Tribune*, March 19, 2012, available at http://articles.chicagotribune.com/2012-03-19/classified/ct-met-getting-around-0319-20120319_1_colgan-air-flight-pilot-error-airline-jobs.

Hill, R.G., Sears, L.M., Melanson, S.W. 2013. 4000 clicks: a productivity analysis of electronic medical records in a community hospital ED. *American Journal of Emergency Medicine* **31**(11):1591–4.

Hill, E.M., Turner, E.L., Martin, R.M., Donovan, J.L. 2013. "Let's get the best quality research we can": public awareness and acceptance of consent to use existing data in health research: a systematic review and qualitative study. *BMC Medical Research Methodology* **13**:72, available at www.biomedcentral.com/1471-2288/13/72.

Hiller, K.M., Stoneking, L., Min, A., Rhodes, S.M. 2013. Syndromic surveillance for influenza in the emergency department – a systematic review. *PLoS One* **8**(9):e73832.

Hippocrates. 1983. *Hippocratic Writings.* Lloyd, G.E.R., ed., Chadwisk, J., Mann, W.N., trans. London: Penguin.

Hirsch, M.D. 2015. Docs to ONC: Change the EHR certification process. *FierceEMR*, January 22, available at www.fierceemr.com/story/docs-onc-change-ehr-certification-process/2015-01-22.

Hirschtick, R.E. 2006. A piece of my mind. Copy-and-paste. *Journal of the American Medical Association* 24;**295**(20):2335–6.

Hochachka, W.M., Fink, D., Hutchinson, R.A., Sheldon, D., Wong, W.K., Kelling, S. 2012. Data-intensive science applied to broad-scale citizen science. *Trends in Ecology & Evolution* **27**(2):130–7.

Hodge, J.G., Gostin, L.O. 2004. *Public Health Practice vs. Research –A Report for Public Health Practitioners Including Cases and Guidance for Making Distinctions.* Atlanta, GA: Council of State and Territorial Epidemiologists.

Hoffman, S., Podgurski, A. 2012. Drug-drug interaction alerts: emphasizing the evidence. *St. Louis University Journal of Health Law & Policy* **5**:298–309.

Holzemer, W.L., Uys, L.R., Chirwa, M.L., Greeff, M., Makoae, L.N., Kohi, T.W., Dlamini, P.S., Stewart, A.L., Mullan, J., Phetlhu, R.D., Wantland, D., Durrheim, K. 2007. Validation of the HIV/AIDS Stigma Instrument – PLWA (HASI-P). *AIDS Care* **19**(8):1002–12.

Hood, L., Lovejoy, J.C., Price, N.D. 2015. Integrating big data and actionable health coaching to optimize wellness. *BMC Medicine* **13**(1):4.

Horsky, J., Schiff, G.D., Johnston, D., Mercincavage, L., Bell, D., Middleton, B. 2012. Interface design principles for usable decision support: a targeted review of best practices for clinical prescribing interventions. *Journal of Biomedical Informatics* **45**(6):1202–16.

Hosking, G. 2014. *Trust: A History.* Oxford: Oxford University Press.

Househ, M., Borycki, E., Kushniruk, A. 2014. Empowering patients through social media: the benefits and challenges. *Health Informatics Journal* **20**(1):50–8.

Howard, A.W. 2002. Automobile restraints for children: a review for clinicians. *Canadian Medical Association Journal* **167**(7):769–73.

Howe, D., Costanzo, M., Fey, P., Gojobori, T., Hannick, L., Hide, W., Hill, D.P., Kania, R., Schaeffer, M., St Pierre, S., Twigger, S., White, O., Rhee, S.Y. 2008. Big data: The future of biocuration. *Nature* 455:47–50.

Hripcsak, G., Bloomrosen, M., FlatelyBrennan, P., Chute, C.G., Cimino, J., Detmer, D.E., Edmunds, M., Embi, P.J., Goldstein, M.M., Hammond, W.E., Keenan, G.M., Labkoff, S., Murphy, S., Safran, C., Speedie, S., Strasberg, H., Temple, F., Wilcox, A.B. 2014. Health data use, stewardship, and governance: ongoing gaps and challenges: a report from AMIA's 2012 Health Policy Meeting. *Journal of the American Medical Informatics Association* 21:204–11.

Hustinx, P. 2010. Privacy by design: delivering the promises. *Identity in the Information Society* 3(2):253–55.

Illman, J. 2000. WHO's plan to police health websites rejected. *BMJ* 321:1308.

Institute of Medicine. 2001. *Preserving Public Trust: Accreditation and Human Research Participant Protection Programs.* Washington, DC: National Academies Press.

Institute of Medicine. 2011. *Digital Infrastructure for the Learning Health System: The Foundation for Continuous Improvement in Health and Health Care: Workshop Series Summary.* Washington, DC: The National Academies Press.

Institute of Medicine. 2012. *Health IT and Patient Safety: Building Safer Systems for Better Care.* Washington, DC: The National Academies Press.

Ioannidis, J.P. 2005. Why most published research findings are false. *PLoS Medicine* 2(8):e124.

Ioannidis, J.P. 2014. How to make more published research true. *PLoS Medicine* 11(10): e1001747.

Isidore of Seville. 2013. *Isidore of Seville's Etymologies: the complete translation of Isidori Hispalensis Episcopi Etymologiarum sive Originum Libri.* Throop, P., trans. Charlotte, VT: MedievalMS.

Jackson, G.L., Powers, B.J., Chatterjee, R., Bettger, J.P., Kemper, A.R., Hasselblad, V., Dolor, R.J., Irvine, R.J., Heidenfelder, B.L., Kendrick, A.S., Gray, R., Williams, J.W. 2013. Improving patient care. The patient centered medical home. A Systematic Review. *Annals of Internal Medicine* 158 (3):169–78.

Jain, S.H. 2009. Practicing medicine in the age of Facebook. *New England Journal of Medicine* 361(7):649–51.

JASON. 2014. A Robust Health Data Infrastructure. Prepared for the US Agency for Healthcare Research and Quality, AHRQ Publication No. 14-0041-EF. McLean, VA: MITRE Corporation, available at http://healthit.gov/sites/default/files/pt p13-700hhs_white.pdf.

Jecker, N.S., Schneiderman, L.J. 1993. Medical futility: the duty not to treat. *Cambridge Quarterly of Health Care Ethics* 2:151–9.

Jennings, B. 2006. The politics of end-of-life decision-making: computerised decision-support tools, physicians' jurisdiction and morality. *Sociology of Health & Illness* 28 (3):350–75.

Jha, A.K., Classen, D.C. 2011.Getting moving on patient safety – harnessing electronic data for safer care. *New England Journal of Medicine* 365(19):1756–8.

Joe, J., Demiris, G. 2013. Older adults and mobile phones for health: a review. *Journal of Biomedical Informatics* 46(5):947–54.

Johnson, D.G. 2006. Computer systems: moral entities but not moral agents. *Ethics and Information Technology* 8:195–204.

Johnson, D.G. 2009. *Computer Ethics.* 4th edn. Upper Saddle River, NJ: Pearson Education.

Johnson, E.J., Goldstein, D. 2003. Do defaults save lives? *Science* 302(5649):1338–9.

Johnson, K.B. 2010. Project Health Design: advancing the vision of consumer-clinician-computer collaborations. *Journal of Biomedical Informatics* 43(5 Suppl):S1–2.

Jonas, H. 1984. *The Imperative of Responsibility. In search of an Ethics for the Technological Age.* Chicago: The University of Chicago Press.

Jonsen, A.R. 1998. *The Birth of Bioethics.* Oxford: Oxford University Press.

Kaplan, B., Shaw, N.T. 2004. Future directions in evaluation research: people, organizational, and social issues. *Methods of Information in Medicine* 43(3):215–31.

Kass, N.E., Faden, R. R., Goodman, S. N., Pronovost, P., Tunis, S., Beauchamp, T. L. 2013. The research-treatment distinction: A problematic approach for determining which activities should have ethical oversight. *Hastings Center Report* 43(S1):S4–S15.

Katz, R.V., Green, B.L., Kressin, N.R., Kegeles, S. S., Wang, M.Q., James, S.A., Russell, S.L., Claudio, C., McCallum, J.M. 2008. The legacy of the Tuskegee Syphilis Study: assessing its impact on willingness to participate in biomedical studies. *Journal of Health Care for the Poor and Underserved* (4):1168–80.

Kawamoto, K., Houlihan, C.A., Balas, E.A., Lobach, D.F. 2005. Improving clinical practice using clinical decision support systems: a systematic review of trials to identify features critical to success. *BMJ* 330(7494):765.

Kaye, J. 2012. The tension between data sharing and the protection of privacy in genomics research. *Annual Review of Genomics and Human Genetics* 13:415–31.

Kho, A.N., Rasmussen, L.V., Connolly, J.J., Peissig, P.L., Starren, J., Hakonarson, H., Hayes, M.G. 2013. Practical challenges in integrating genomic data into the electronic health record. *Genetics in Medicine* 15(10):772–8.

Khum, H.D., Ahalt, S. 2013. Privacy-by-design: Understanding data access models for secondary data. *AMIA Joint Summits on Translational Science Proceedings*, March 18:126–30, available at www.ncbi.nlm.nih.gov/pmc/articles/PMC3845756/.

Kim, S., Kim, W., Park, R.W. 2011. A comparison of intensive care unit mortality prediction models through the use of data mining techniques. *Healthcare Informatics Research* 17(4):232–43.

King, A.C., Bickmore, T.W., Campero, M.I., Pruitt, L.A., Yin, J.L. 2013. Employing virtual advisors in preventive care for underserved communities: results from the COMPASS study. *Journal of Health Communication* 18 (12):1449–64.

Kluge, E.-H. 2001. *The Ethics of Electronic Patient Records*. New York: Peter Lang.

Knaus, W.A. 1993. Ethical implications of risk stratification in the acute care setting. *Cambridge Quarterly of Healthcare Ethics* 2:193–6.

Knaus, W.A. 2002. APACHE 1978–2001: the development of a quality assurance system based on prognosis: milestones and personal reflections. *Archives of Surgery* 137(1):37–41.

Knaus, W.A., Draper, E.A., Wagner, D.P., Zimmerman, J.E. 1985. APACHE II: a severity of disease classification system. *Critical Care Medicine* 13:818–29.

Knaus, W.A., Draper, E.A., Wagner, D.P., Zimmerman, J.E. 1986. An evaluation of outcome from intensive care in major medical centers. *Annals of Internal Medicine* 104:410–18.

Knaus, W.A., Wagner, D.P., Lynn, J. 1991. Short-term mortality predictions for critically ill hospitalized adults: science and ethics. *Science* 254:389–94.

Knaus, W.A., Zimmerman, J.E., Wagner, D.P., Draper, E.A., Lawrence, D.E. 1981. APACHE – acute physiology and chronic health evaluation: a physiologically based classification system. *Critical Care Medicine* (9):591–7.

Kobeissy, F.H., Gulbakan, B., Alawieh, A., Karam, P., Zhang, Z., Guingab-Cagmat, J.D., Mondello, S., Tan, W., Anagli, J., Wang, K. 2014. Post-genomics nanotechnology is gaining momentum: nanoproteomics and applications in life sciences. *OMICS* 18(2):111–31.

Kohane, I.S. 2013. Secondary use of health information: are we asking the right question? *JAMA Internal Medicine* 173(19):1806–7.

Kohn, L.T., Corrigan, J.M., Donaldson, M.S., eds. 1999. *To Err Is Human: Building a Safer Health System*. Washington, DC: National Academy Press.

Koppel, R., Kreda, D. 2009. Health care information technology vendors' "hold harmless" clause: implications for patients and clinicians. *Journal of the American Medical Association* 301(12):1276–78.

Koppel, R., Metlay, J.P., Cohen, A., Abaluck, B., Localio, A.R., Kimmel, S.E., Strom, B.L. 2005. Role of computerized physician order entry systems in facilitating medication errors. *Journal of the American Medical Association* 293(10):1197–203.

Kraemer Diaz, A.E., Spears Johnson, C.R., Arcury, T.A. 2015. Perceptions that influence the maintenance of scientific integrity in community-based participatory research. *Health, Education & Behavior*, January 14. pii: 1090198114560016.

Kramer, A.A., Higgins, T.L., Zimmerman, J.E. 2013. The association between ICU readmission rate and patient outcomes. *Critical Care Medicine* 41(1):24–33.

Kramer, A.D.I., Guillory, J.E., Hancock, J.T. 2014. Experimental evidence of massive-scale emotional contagion through social networks. *Proceedings of the National Academy of Sciences* 111:8788–90.

Kuhn, T., Basch, P., Barr, M., Yackel, T., for the Medical Informatics Committee of the American College of Physicians. 2015. Clinical documentation in the 21st century: Executive summary of a policy position paper from the American College of Physicians. *Annals of Internal Medicine* 162(2):301–3.

Kullo, I.J., Haddad, R., Prows, C.A., Holm, I., Sanderson, S.C., Garrison, N.A., Sharp, R.R., Smith, M.E., Kuivaniemi, H., Bottinger, E.P., Connolly, J.J., Keating, B.J., McCarty, C.A., Williams, M.S., Jarvik, G.P. 2014. Return of results in the genomic medicine projects of the eMERGE network. *Frontiers in Genetics* 5:50.

Kumar, A., Asaf, B.B. 2015. Robotic thoracic surgery: The state of the art. *Journal of Minimal Access Surgery* 11(1):60–7.

Kush, R., Goldman, M. 2014. Fostering responsible data sharing through standards. *New England Journal of Medicine* 370:2163–5.

Laennec, R.T.H. 1821. *A Treatise on the Diseases of the Chest, in Which They Are Described According to Their Anatomical Characters, and Their Diagnosis Established on a New Principle by Means of Acoustick Instruments.* Forbes, J., trans. London: T. and G. Underwood. [Full text available via The Gerstein Science Information Centre at the University of Toronto at http://archive.org/stream/treatiseondiseas00laen/treatiseondi seas00laen_djvu.txt.]

Lainer, M., Mann, E., Sönnichsen, A. 2013. Information technology interventions to improve medication safety in primary care: a systematic review. *International Journal for Quality in Heath Care* 25(5):590–8.

Lane, W.A. 1936. What the mouth reveals. *New Health* 11:34–5.

Lane J., Schur, C. 2010. Balancing access to health data and privacy: a review of the issues and approaches for the future. *Health Services Research* 45(5 Pt 2):1456–67.

Laranjo, L., Arguel, A., Neves, A.L., Gallagher, A.M., Kaplan, R., Mortimer, N., Mendes, G.A., Lau, A.Y. 2014. The influence of social networking sites on health behavior change: a systematic review and meta-analysis. *Journal of the American Medical Informatics Association*, July 8. pii: amiajnl-2014-002841.

Lau, A. 2009. What are repeatability and reproducibility? Part 1: A DO2 viewpoint for laboratories. ASTM Standardization News March/April, available at www.astm.org/SN EWS/MA_2009/datapoints_ma09.html.

Lau, K.H. 2014. Computer-based teaching module design: principles derived from learning theories. *Medical Education* 48(3):247–54.

Law Commission. 1996. Privity of contract: Contracts for the benefit of third parties LC242, available at http://lawcommission.justice.gov.uk/docs/lc242_privity_of_contract_for_the_benefit_of_third_parties.pdf.

Law, L.M., Wason, J.M. 2014. Design of telehealth trials – Introducing adaptive approaches. *International Journal of Medical Informatics* 83(12):870–80.

Lee, L.M. 2014. Health information in the background: justifying public health surveillance without patient consent. In Pimple, K.D., ed., *Emerging Pervasive Information and Communication Technologies (PICT): Ethical Challenges, Opportunities and Safeguards.* Dordrecht: Springer, 39–53.

Lee, L.M., Gostin, L.O. 2009. Ethical collection, storage, and use of public health data: A proposal for a national privacy protection. *Journal of the American Medical Association* 302(1):82–4.

Lee, L.M., Hellig, C.M., White, A. 2012. Ethical justification for conducting public health surveillance without patient consent. *American Journal of Public Health* 102(1):38–44.

Leviss, J., ed. 2013. *HIT or Miss: Lessons Learned from Health Information Technology Implementations.* 2nd edn. Chicago: AHIMA.

Lewandowsky, S., Gignac, G.E., Oberauer, K. 2013. The role of conspiracist ideation and worldviews in predicting rejection of science. *PLoS One* 8(10):e75637.

Lim, J.L., Yih, Y., Gichunge, C., Tierney, W.M., Le, T.H., Zhang, J., Lawley, M.A, Petersen, T.J., Mamlin, J.J. 2009. The AMPATH Nutritional Information System: designing a food distribution electronic record system in rural Kenya. *Journal of the American Medical Informatics Association* 16(6):882–8.

Lin, P., Abney, K., Bekey, G.A., eds. 2012. *Robot Ethics: The Ethical and Social Implications of Robots.* Cambridge, MA: MIT Press.

Lorsch, J.R., Collins, F.S., Lippincott-Schwartz, J. 2014. Fixing problems with cell lines. *Science* 346(6216):1452–3

Louis, P.C.A. 1834. *Essay on Clinical Instruction.* Martin, P., trans. London: S. Highley. (Cited in E.J. Huth and T.J. Murray, eds., *Medicine in Quotations: Views of Health and Disease Through the Ages.* Philadelphia: American College of Physicians.)

Louis, P.C.A. 1835/1960. Research on the effect of blood-letting in several inflammatory maladies. Translation of an article by Pierre-Charles-Alexander Louis (*Arch. gen. Méd.* 321–336, 1835), with introduction. Gaines, W.J., Langford, H.G., trans. *Archives of Internal Medicine* **106**(4):571–9. doi:10.1001/archinte.1960.03820040109009.

Louis, P.C.A. 1836. *Researches on the Effects of Bloodletting in Some Inflammatory Diseases, and on the Influence of Tartarized Antimony and Vesication in Pneumonitis.* Putnam, C.G., trans. Boston: Hilliard, Gray & Co. Full text available via The Gerstein Science Information Centre at the University of Toronto at https://archive.org/details/researchesoneffe00louiuoft.

Lown, B.A., Rodriguez, D. 2012. Lost in translation? How electronic health records structure communication, relationships, and meaning. *Academic Medicine* **87**(4):392–4.

Lowy, J. 2011. Automation in the air dulls pilot skill. *The Associated Press*, available at http://news.yahoo.com/ap-impact-automation-air-dulls-pilot-skill-070507795.html.

Lowry, S.Z., Ramaiah, M., Patterson, E.S., Latkany, P., Brick, D., Gibbons, M.C. 2015. *Integrating Electronic Health Records into Clinical Workflow: An Application of Human Factors Modeling Methods to Obstetrics and Gynecology and Ophthalmology.* Washington, DC: National Institute of Standards and Technology (NISTIR 8042), available at http://nvlpubs.nist.gov/nistpubs/ir/2015/NIST.IR.8042.pdf.

Luce, J.M., Wachter, R.M. 1994. The ethical appropriateness of using prognostic scoring systems in clinical management. *Critical Care Clinics* **10**:229–41.

Mack, E.H., Wheeler, D.S., Embi, P.J. 2009. Clinical decision support systems in the pediatric intensive care unit. *Pediatric Critical Care Medicine* **10**(1):23–8.

Mackey, T.K., Liang, B.A., Attaran, A., Kohler, J.C. 2013. Ensuring the future of health information online. *Lancet* **382** (9902):1404.

Mackey, T.K., Liang, B.A., Kohler, J.C., Attaran, A. 2014. Health domains for sale: the need for global health Internet governance. *Journal of Medical Internet Research* **16**(3):e62.

Magnello, E. 2011. Vital Statistics: The measurement of public health. In Flood, R., Rice, A., Wilson, R., eds., *Mathematics in Victorian Britain.* Oxford: Oxford University Press, 261–82.

Magrabi, F., Baker, M., Sinha, I., Ong, M.S., Harrison, S., Kidd, M.R., Runciman, W.B., Coiera, E. 2015. Clinical safety of England's national programme for IT: A retrospective analysis of all reported safety events 2005 to 2011. *International Journal of Medical Informatics* **84**(3):198–206.

Malin, B. 2011. HIPAA and a learning healthcare system. In Institute of Medicine, *Digital Infrastructure for the Learning Health System: The Foundation for Continuous Improvement in Health and Health Care: Workshop Series Summary.* Washington, DC: The National Academies Press, 157–61.

Malin, B., Loukides, G., Benitez, K., Clayton, E.W. 2011. Identifiability in biobanks: models, measures, and mitigation strategies. *Human Genetics* **130**:383–92.

Malin, B., Sweeney, L. 2004. How (not) to protect genomic data privacy in a distributed network: using trail re-identification to evaluate and design anonymity protection systems *Journal of Biomedical Informatics* **37**:179–92.

Maloni, J.M, Brown, M.E. 2006. Corporate social responsibility in the supply chain: An application in the food industry. *Journal of Business Ethics*, **68**:35–52.

Mamykina, L., Vawdrey, D.K., Stetson, P.D., Zheng, K., Hripcsak, G. 2012. Clinical documentation: composition or synthesis? *Journal of the American Medical Informatics Association* **19**:1025–31.

Mandl, K.D., Kohane, I.S. 2008. Tectonic shifts in the health information economy. *New England Journal of Medicine* **358**:1732–7.

Manhal-Baugus, M. 2001. E-therapy: practical, ethical, and legal issues. *CyberPsychology & Behavior* **4**(5):551–63.

Markle Foundation. 2006. *Connecting Americans to Their Health Care: A Common Framework for Networked Personal Health*

Information. New York: Markle Foundation, available at www.markle.org.

Markle Foundation. 2008. *Americans Overwhelmingly Believe Electronic Personal Health Records Could Improve Their Health (based on a survey by Prof. A.F. Westin)*. New York: Markle Foundation, available at www.markle.org.

Marquard, J.L., Brennan, P.F. 2009. Crying wolf: Consumers may be more willing to share medication information than policymakers think. *Journal of Health Information Management* 23(2):26–32.

McCorduck, P. 2004. *Machines Who Think: A Personal Inquiry into the History and Prospects of Artificial Intelligence*. 2nd edn. London: CRC Press.

McCoy, A.B., Melton, G.B., Wright, A., Sittig, D. F. 2013. Clinical decision support for colon and rectal surgery: an overview. *Clinics in Colon and Rectal Surgery* 26(1):23–30.

McCoy, A.B., Waitman, L.R., Lewis, J.B., Wright, J.A., Choma, D.P., Miller, R.A., Peterson, J.F. 2012. A framework for evaluating the appropriateness of clinical decision support alerts and responses. *Journal of the American Medical Informatics Association* 19(3):346–52.

McDaid, D., Park, A-L. 2011. Online Health: Untangling the Web. BUPA Health Pulse 2010. London School of Economics and British United Provident Association (BUPA), available at www.bupa.com.au/static files/Bupa/HealthAndWellness/MediaFiles/PDF/LSE_Report_Online_Health.pdf.

McDonald, C.J. 1976. Protocol-based computer reminders, the quality of care and the non-perfectability of man. *New England Journal of Medicine* 295(24):1351–5.

McEwen, J.E., Boyer, J.T., Sun, K.Y., Rothenberg, K.H., Lockhart, N.C., Guyer, M.S. 2014. The ethical, legal, and social implications program of the national human genome research institute: reflections on an ongoing experiment. *Annual Review of Genomics and Human Genetics* 15:481–505.

McGraw, D. 2011. Policies and practices to build public trust. In Institute of Medicine, *Digital Infrastructure for the Learning Health System: The Foundation for Continuous Improvement in Health and Health Care: Workshop Series Summary*. Washington, DC: The National Academies Press, 155–7.

Meeks, D.W., Smith, M.W., Taylor, L., Sittig, D. F., Scott, J.M., Singh, H. 2014. An analysis of electronic health record-related patient safety concerns. *Journal of the American Medical Informatics Association* 21(6):1053–59.

Menon, S., Smith, M.W., Sittig, D.F., Petersen, N. J., Hysong, S.J., Espadas, D., Modi, V., Singh, H. 2014. How context affects electronic health record-based test result follow-up: a mixed-methods evaluation. *BMJ Open* 4(11): e005985.

Meslin, E.M., Alpert, S.A., Carroll, A.E., Odell, J. D., Tierney, W.M., Schwartz, P.H. 2013. Giving patients granular control of personal health information: using an ethics 'Points to Consider' to inform informatics system designers. *International Journal of Medical Informatics* 82(12):1136–43.

Meslin, E.M., Goodman, K.W. 2010. Bank on it: An ethics and policy agenda for biobanks and electronic health records. *Science Progress*, Center for American Progress, http://science progress.org/2010/02/bank-on-it/#_edn25.

Meslin, E.M., Schwartz, P.H. 2014. How bioethics principles can aid design of electronic health records to accommodate patient granular control. *Journal of General Internal Medicine* 30(Suppl 1):S3–6.

Meyers, D., Quinn, M., Clancy, C.M. 2010. *Health Information Technology: Turning the Patient-Centered Medical Home from Concept to Reality*. Rockville, MD: Agency for Healthcare Research and Quality, available at www.ahrq.gov/news/newsroom/comment aries/pcmh-concept-to-reality.html.

Middleton, B., Bloomrosen, M., Dente, M.A., Hashmat, B., Koppel, R., Overhage, J.M., Payne, T.H., Rosenbloom, S.T., Weaver, C., Zhang, J. 2013. Enhancing patient safety and quality of care by improving the usability of electronic health record systems: recommendations from AMIA. *Journal of the American Medical Informatics Association* 20:e2–e8.

Mill, J.S. 1956 (1859). *On Liberty*. Indianapolis: The Bobbs-Merrill Company.

Miller, R.A. 1990. Why the standard view is standard: people, not machines, understand patients' problems. *Journal of Medicine and Philosophy* 15:581–91.

Miller, R.A., Gardner, R.M. 1997a. Summary recommendations for the responsible monitoring and regulation of clinical software systems. *Annals of Internal Medicine* 127(9):842–5.

Miller, R.A., Gardner, R.M. 1997b. Recommendations for responsible monitoring and regulation of clinical software systems. *Journal of the American Medical Informatics Association* 4:442–57.

Miller, R.A., Schaffner, K.F., Meisel, A. 1985. Ethical and legal issues related to the use of computer programs in clinical medicine. *Annals of Internal Medicine* 102:529–36.

Moor, J.H. 1979. Are there decisions computers should never make? *Nature and System* 1:217–29.

Moore, D.A., Tetlock, P.E., Tanlu, L., Bazerman, M.H. 2006. Conflict of interest and the case of auditor independence: Moral seduction and strategic issue cycling. *Academy of Management Review* 31(1):10–29.

Moreno, R., Afonso, S. 2006. Ethical, legal and organizational issues in the ICU: prediction of outcome. *Current Opinions in Critical Care* 12(6):619–23.

Morens, D.M. 1999. Death of a president. *New England Journal of Medicine* 341:1845–50.

Morris, G., Farnum, G., Afzal, S., Robinson, C., Greene, J., Coughlin, C. 2014. Patient Identification and Matching Final Report. Office of the National Coordinator for Health Information Technology, contract HHSP233201300029C, available at www.healthit.gov/sites/default/files/patient_identification_matching_final_report.pdf.

Mushiaki, S. 2013. Ethica ex machina: issues in roboethics. *Journal international de bioéthique* 24(4):17–26, 176–7.

Nanji, K.C., Slight, S.P., Seger, D.L., Cho. I., Fiskio, J.M., Redden, L.M., Volk, L.A., Bates, D.W. 2014. Overrides of medication-related clinical decision support alerts in outpatients. *Journal of the American Medical Informatics Association* 21(3):487–91.

National Bioethics Advisory Commission. 2001. *Ethical and Policy Issues in International Research: Clinical Trials in Developing Countries.* Vol. 1. Bethesda, MD: National Bioethics Advisory Commission.

National Research Council. 1997. *For the Record: Protecting Electronic Health Information.* Washington, DC: National Academy Press.

Nazi, K.M., Hogan, T.P., Wagner, T.H., McInnes, D.K., Smith, B.M., Haggstrom, D., Chumbler, N.R., Gifford, A.L., Charters, K.G., Saleem, J.J., Weingardt, K.R., Fischetti, L.F., Weaver, F.M. 2010. Embracing a health services research perspective on personal health records: Lessons learned from the VA My HealtheVet system. *Journal of General Internal Medicine* 25(Suppl 1):62–7.

Newman-Toker, D.E., Pronovost, P.J. 2009. Diagnostic errors–the next frontier for patient safety. *Journal of the American Medical Association* 301:1060–2.

Nissenbaum, H. 1994. Computing and accountability. *Communications of the Association for Computing Machinery* 37(1):72–80.

Nissenbaum, H. 2000. Values in computer system design: Bias and autonomy. In Collste, G., ed., *Ethics in the Age of Information Technology.* Studies in Applied Ethics 7. Linköping: Centre for Applied Ethics, 59–69.

Noorman, M. 2014. Computing and moral responsibility. In Zalta, E.N., ed., *The Stanford Encyclopedia of Philosophy* (Summer 2014 edn.), available at http://plato.stanford.edu/archives/sum2014/entries/computing-responsibility/.

Nuffield Council on Bioethics. 2015. *The Collection, Linking and Use of Data in Biomedical Research and Health Care: Ethical Issues.* London: Nuffield Council on Bioethics, available at http://nuffieldbioethics.org/wp-content/uploads/Biological_and_health_data_web.pdf.

Nutton, V. 1996. The rise of medicine. In Porter, R., ed., *The Cambridge Illustrated History of Medicine.* Cambridge: Cambridge University Press, 52–81.

Office for National Statistics. 2013. Internet Access – Households and Individuals, 2013, available at www.ons.gov.uk/ons/dcp171778_322713.pdf.

Office of Technology Assessment (OTA). 1993a. *Report Brief: Protecting Privacy in Computerized Medical Information.* Washington, DC: US Government Printing Office.

Office of Technology Assessment (OTA). 1993b. *Protecting Privacy in Computerized Medical Information.* Washington, DC: US Government Printing Office (OTA-TCT-576).

Or, C.K., Tao, D. 2014. Does the use of consumer health information technology improve outcomes in the patient self-management of diabetes? A meta-analysis and narrative review of randomized controlled trials.

International Journal of Medical Informatics 83(5):320–9.

Orr, R.D., Pang, N., Pellegrino, E.D., Siegler, M. 1997. Use of the Hippocratic Oath: a review of twentieth century practice and a content analysis of oaths administered in medical schools in the US and Canada in 1993. *Journal of Clinical Ethics* 8(4):377–88.

Overby, C.L., Tarczy-Hornoch, P., Kalet, I.J., Thummel, K.E., Smith, J.W., Del Fiol, G., Fenstermacher, D., Devine, E.B. 2012. Developing a Prototype system for integrating pharmacogenomics findings into clinical practice. *Journal of Personalized Medicine* 2, 241–56.

Ozoliņa, Z., Mitcham, C., Stilgoe, J., Andanda, P., Kaiser, M., Nielsen, L., Stehr, N., Qiu, R.-Z. 2009. Global Governance of Science: Report of the Expert Group on Global Governance of Science to the Science, Economy and Society Directorate, Directorate-General for Research, European Commission, EUR23616 EN, available at http://ec.europa.eu/research/swafs/pdf/pub_archive/global-governance-020609_en.pdf.

Palmer, B. 2014. Jonas Salk: Good at virology, bad at economics. *Slate*, April 13, 2014, available at www.slate.com/articles/technology/history_of_innovation/2014/04/the_real_reasons_jonas_salk_didn_t_patent_the_polio_vaccine.html.

Palmer, V. 1983. Why privity entered tort – an historical reexamination of *Winterbottom v. Wright. The American Journal of Legal History* 27(1):85–98.

Palmer, V. 1992. *The Paths to Privity: A History of Third Party Beneficiary Contracts at English Law*. San Francisco: Austin & Winfield.

Patel, M.S., Asch, D.A., Volpp, K.G. 2015. Wearable devices as facilitators, not drivers, of health behavior change. *Journal of the American Medical Association* 323(5):459–60.

Patel, V., Barker, W., Siminerio, E. 2014. *Individuals' Access and Use of their Online Medical Record Nationwide*. ONC Data Brief No. 2. Washington, DC: Office of the National Coordinator for Health Information Technology, available at www.healthit.gov/sites/default/files/consumeraccessdatabrief_9_10_14.pdf.

Pauker, S.G., Kassirer, J.P. 1981. Clinical decision analysis by personal computer. *Archives of Internal Medicine* 141(13):1831–7.

Pearson, S.-A., Moxey, A., Robertson, J., Hains, I., Williamson, M., Reeve, J., Newby, D. 2009. Do computerised clinical decision support systems for prescribing change practice? A systematic review of the literature (1990–2007). *BMC Health Services Research* 9:154.

Penson, R.T., Kyriakou, H., Zuckerman, D., Chabner, B.A., Lynch, T.J. 2006. Teams: communication in multidisciplinary care. *Oncologist* 11(5):520–526.

Perry, J.E., Cox, D., Cox, A.D. 2014. Trust and transparency: patient perceptions of physicians' financial relationships with pharmaceutical companies. *Journal of Law, Medicine, and Ethics* 42(4):475–91.

Petersen, C., DeMuro, P. 2015. Legal and regulatory considerations associated with use of patient-generated health data from social media and mobile health (mHealth) devices. *Applied Clinical Informatics* 6(1):16–26.

Petersen, C., DeMuro, P., Goodman, K.W., Kaplan, B. 2013. Sorrell v. IMS Health: issues and opportunities for informaticians. *Journal of the American Medical Informatics Association* 20(1):35–7.

Phansalkar, S., Zachariah, M., Seidling, H.M., Mendes, C., Volk, L., Bates, D.W. 2014. Evaluation of medication alerts in electronic health records for compliance with human factors principles. *Journal of the American Medical Informatics Association* 21(e2):e332–40.

Phelps, R.G., Taylor, J., Simpson, K., Samuel, J., Turner, A.N. 2014. Patients' continuing use of an online health record: a quantitative evaluation of 14,000 patient years of access data. *Journal of Medical Internet Research* 16 (10):e241.

Picciano, K.S., Goodman, K.W. 2014. *Clinical Decision Support Systems: A Survey of Some Legal and Ethical Implications*. Working Papers in Bioethics. Miami: University of Miami Bioethics Program.

Pimple, K.D. 2014. Introduction: The Impact, Benefits, and Hazards of PICT. In Pimple, K.D., ed., *Emerging Pervasive Information and Communication Technologies (PICT): Ethical Challenges, Opportunities and Safeguards*. Dordrecht: Springer, 1–12.

Pinker, S. 2008. The Stupidity of Dignity: Conservative bioethics' latest, most dangerous ploy. *The New Republic*, May 28, available at http://pinker.wjh.harvard.edu/articles/media/The%20Stupidity%20of%20Dignity.htm.

Platt, J., Kardia, S. 2015. Public trust in health information sharing: implications for bio-banking and electronic health record systems. *Journal of Personalized Medicine* **5** (1):3–21.

Popper, K.R. 1959/1980. *The Logic of Scientific Discovery*. London: Hutchinson.

Porter, R. 1992. The rise of medical journalism in Britain to 1800. In Bynum, W.F., Lock, S., and Porter, R., eds., *Medical Journals and Medical Knowledge: Historical Essays*. London and New York: Routledge, 6–28.

Postel, J. 1994. Domain Name System Structure and Delegation. University of Southern California Information Sciences Institute, available at http://tools.ietf.org/pdf/rfc1591.pdf.

Presidential Commission for the Study of Bioethical Issues. 2011. *Moral Science: Protecting Participants in Human Subjects Research*. Washington, DC: Presidential Commission for the Study of Bioethical Issues.

Prinzel, L.J., Pope, A.T., Freeman F.G., 2002. Physiological self-regulation and adaptive automation. *International Journal of Aviation Psychology* 12(2):179–96.

Rachels, J. 1975. Why is privacy important? *Philosophy & Public Affairs* 4(4):323–33.

Radley, D.C., Wasserman, M.R., Olsho, L.E., Shoemaker, S.J., Spranca, M.D., Bradshaw, B. 2013. Reduction in medication errors in hospitals due to adoption of computerized provider order entry systems. *Journal of the American Medical Informatics Association* **20** (3):470–6.

Reiser, S.J. 1991.The clinical record in medicine. Part 1: Learning from cases. *Annals of Internal Medicine* 114:902–7.

Reynolds, T., Kong, M.-L. 2011. Learning without patients: How far can medical simulation replace clinical experience? *BMJ* 342:83–4.

Rosenthal, T.C. 2008. The medical home: Growing evidence to support a new approach to primary care. *Journal of the American Board of Family Medicine* 21(5):427–40.

Rotich, J.K., Hannan, T.J., Smith, F.E., Bii, J., Odero, W.W., Vu, N., Mamlin, B.W., Mamlin, J.J., Einterz, R.M., Tierney, W.M. 2003. Installing and implementing a computer-based patient record system in sub-Saharan Africa: the Mosoriot Medical Record System. *Journal of the American Medical Informatics Association* **10** (4):295–303.

Ridgely, M.S., Greenberg, M.D. 2012. Too many alerts, too much liability: sorting through the malpratice implications of drug-drug interaction clinical decision support. *St. Louis University Journal of Health Law & Policy* 5:257–96.

Rogers, J.A. 2015. Electronics for the human body. *Journal of the American Medical Association* 313(6):561–2.

Ross, M.K., Wei, W., Ohno-Machado, L. 2014. "Big data" and the electronic health record. *Yearbook of Medical Informatics* 9(1):97–104.

Rothstein, M.S. 2010. The Hippocratic bargain and health information technology. *Journal of Law, Medicine & Ethics* 38(1):7–13.

Rubel, A. 2012. Justifying public health surveillance: basic interests, unreasonable exercise, and privacy. *Kennedy Institute of Ethics Journal* 22(1):1–33.

Rubin, D.L., Lewis, S.E., Mungall, C.J., Misra, S., Westerfield, M., Ashburner, M., Sim, I., Chute, C.G., Solbrig, H., Storey, M.A., Smith, B., Day-Richter, J., Noy, N.F., Musen, M.A. 2006. National Center for Biomedical Ontology: advancing biomedicine through structured organization of scientific knowledge. *OMICS* 10(2):185–98.

Russell, A.L. 2014. *Open Standards and the Digital Age: History, Ideology, and Networks*. New York: Cambridge University Press.

Ryan, T., Chester, A., Reece, J., Xenos, S. 2014. The uses and abuses of Facebook: A review of Facebook addiction. *Journal of Behavioral Addictions* 3(3):133–48.

Sackett, D.L., Straus, S.E., Richardson, W.S., Rosenberg, W., Haynes, R.B. 2000. *Evidence-Based Medicine: How to Practice and Teach EBM*. 2nd edn. Edinburgh: Churchill Livingstone.

Sadegh-Zadeh, K. 2012. *Handbook of Analytic Philosophy of Medicine*. Dordrecht: Springer.

Sadler, N.L., Sadler, A.M. 2012. Can Social Media Increase Transplant Donation and Save Lives? Science and Society, Hastings Center Bioethics Forum, available at www.thehastingscenter.org/Bioethicsforum/Post.aspx?id=5950.

Safran, C., Bloomrosen, M., Hammond, W.E., Labkoff, S., Markel-Fox, S., Tang, P.C.,

Detmer, D.E. 2007. Toward a national framework for the secondary use of health data: an American Medical Informatics Association White Paper. *Journal of the American Medical Informatics Association* 14(1):1–9.

Salathé, M., Freifeld, C.C., Mekaru, S.R., Tomasulo, A.F., Brownstein, J.S. 2013. Influenza A (H7N9) and the importance of digital epidemiology. *New England Journal of Medicine* 369:401–4.

Schneiderman, L.J., Jecker, N.S. 1995. *Wrong Medicine: Doctors, Patients, and Futile Treatment.* Baltimore: Johns Hopkins University Press.

Scullard, P., Peacock, C., Davies, P. 2010. Googling children's health: reliability of medical advice on the internet. *Archives of Disease in Childhood* 95(8):580–2.

Seck, M.D., Evans, D.D. 2004. *Major U.S. Cities Using National Standard Fire Hydrants, One Century After the Great Baltimore Fire.* Gaithersburg, MD: National Institute of Standards and Technology (NISTIR 7158), available at www.fire.nist.gov/bfrlpubs/fire04/PDF/f04095.pdf.

Shannon, G.W., Buker, C.M. 2010. Determining accessibility to dermatologists and teledermatology locations in Kentucky: demonstration of an innovative geographic information systems approach. *Telemedicine Journal and e-Health* 16(6):670–7.

Sharkey, N., Sharkey, A. 2012. The rights and wrongs of Robot Care. In Lin, P., Abney, K., Bekey, G.A., eds., *Robot Ethics: The Ethical and Social Implications of Robots.* Cambridge, MA: MIT Press, 267–82.

Shaw, G. 1909. *The Doctor's Dilemma: With Preface on Doctors.* New York: Brentano's.

Shaw, J. 2006. Intention in ethics. *Canadian Journal of Philosophy* 36(2):187–223.

Shortliffe, E.H. 1993. Doctors, patients, and computers: Will information technology dehumanize health-care delivery? *Proceedings of the American Philosophical Society* 137(3):390–8.

Shortliffe, E.H. 1994. Dehumanization of patient care: Are computers the problem or the solution? *Journal of the American Medical Informatics Association* 1:76–78.

Shortliffe, E.H. 2011. Demonstrating value to secure trust. In Institute of Medicine, *Digital Infrastructure for the Learning Health System:* *The Foundation for Continuous Improvement in Health and Health Care: Workshop Series Summary.* Washington, DC: The National Academies Press, 151–5.

Shortliffe, E.H., Blois, M.S. 2014. Biomedical informatics: the science and the pragmatics. In Shortliffe, E.H., Cimino, J.J., eds., *Biomedical Informatics: Computer Applications in Health Care and Biomedicine.* 4th edn. New York: Springer, 3–37.

Shortliffe, E.H., Cimino, J.J., eds. 2014. *Biomedical Informatics: Computer Applications in Health Care and Biomedicine.* 4th edn. New York: Springer.

Siegler, E.L. 2010. The evolving medical record. *Annals of Internal Medicine* 153:671–7.

Siegler, E.L., Adelman, R. 2009. Copy and paste: A remediable hazard of electronic health records. *American Journal of Medicine* 122:495–6.

Simon, H.A. 1971. Designing organizations for an information-rich world. In Greenberger, M., ed., *Computers, Communication, and the Public Interest.* Baltimore, MD: The Johns Hopkins Press, 37–52.

Simon, H.A. 1985. Artificial-intelligence approaches to problem solving and clinical diagnosis. In Schaffner, K.F., ed., *Logic of Discovery and Diagnosis in Medicine.* Berkeley: University of California Press, 72–93.

Sims, R. R., Brinkmann, J. 2003. Enron ethics (or culture matters more than codes). *Journal of Business Ethics* 45(3),243–56.

Singer, P. 1972. Famine, affluence, and morality. *Philosophy and Public Affairs* 1(1):229–43.

Slack, W.V. 1989. The computer and the doctor-patient relationship. *M.D. Computing* 6(6):320–1.

Smith, L. 2011. The Kahun Gynaecological Papyrus: ancient Egyptian medicine. *Journal of Family Planning and Reproductive Health Care* 37:54–5.

Smith, L. 2013. The history of contraception. In Briggs, P., Kovacs, G., Guillebaud, J., eds., *Contraception: A Casebook from Menarche to Menopause.* Cambridge: Cambridge University Press, 18–25.

Snapper, J.W. 1998. Responsibility for computer-based decisions in health care. In Goodman, K.W., ed., *Ethics, Computing, and Medicine: Informatics and the Transformation of Health Care.* Cambridge: Cambridge University Press, 43–56.

Snell, K., Starkbaum, J., Lauß, G., Vermeer, A., Helén, I. 2012. From protection of privacy to control of data streams: a focus group study on biobanks in the information society. *Public Health Genomics* 15(5):293–302.

Snyder, L., American College of Physicians Ethics, Professionalism, and Human Rights Committee. 2012. American college of physicians ethics manual: sixth edition. *Annals of Internal Medicine* 156(1 Pt. 2):73–104.

Sommers, B.D., Baicker, K., Epstein, A.M. 2012. Mortality and access to care among adults after state Medicaid expansions. *New England Journal of Medicine* 367:1025–34.

Sorenson, C., Drummond, M. 2014. Improving medical device regulation: the United States and Europe in perspective. *Milbank Quarterly* 92(1):114–50.

Spruill, J.A. 1941. Privity of contract as a requisite for recovery on warranty. *North Carolina Law Review* 19:551–67.

Stangl, A.L., Lloyd, J.K., Brady, L.M., Holland, C.E., Baral, S. 2013. A systematic review of interventions to reduce HIV-related stigma and discrimination from 2002 to 2013: how far have we come? *Journal of the International AIDS Society* 16(3 Suppl. 2):18734.

Stanley, F.J., Meslin, E.M. 2007. Australia needs a better system for health care evaluation. *Medical Journal of Australia* 186:220–1.

Stell, L.K. 2014. Volume-outcome disparities and informed consent: What should surgeons disclose? *Journal of Surgical Oncology*, July 8. doi:10.1002/jso.23718. [Epub ahead of print].

Stevens, J.M. 1975. Gynaecology from ancient Egypt: The papyrus Kahun: A translation of the oldest treatise on gynaecology that has survived from the ancient world. *Medical Journal of Australia* 2(25–26):949–52.

Stroup, D.F., Berkelman, R.L. 1988. History of statistical methods in public health. In Stroup, D.F., Teutsch, S.M., eds., *Statistics in Public Health: Quantitative Approaches to Public Health Problems*. Oxford: Oxford University Press, 1–18.

Sulmasy, D.P., Marx, E.S. 1997. A computerized system for entering orders to limit treatment: implementation and evaluation. *Journal of Clinical Ethics* 8(3):258–63.

Swan, M. 2009. Emerging patient-driven health care models: an examination of health social networks, consumer personalized medicine and quantified self-tracking. *International Journal of Environmental Research and Public Health* 6(2):492–525.

Swan, M. 2012a. Health 2050: The realization of personalized medicine through crowdsourcing, the quantified self, and the participatory biocitizen. *Journal of Personalized Medicine* 2(3):93–118.

Swan, M. 2012b. Crowdsourced health research studies: an important emerging complement to clinical trials in the public health research ecosystem. *Journal of Medical Internet Research* 14(2):e46.

Sweeney, L. 1997. Weaving technology and policy together to maintain confidentiality. *Journal of Law, Medicine and Ethics* 25:98–110.

Szczepaniak, M.C., Goodman, K.W., Wagner, M.W., Hutman, J., Daswani, S. 2006. Advancing organizational integration: negotiation, data use agreements, law, and ethics. In Wagner, M.W., Moore, A.W., Aryel, R.M., eds. *Handbook of Biosurveillance*. Boston: Academic Press, 465–80.

Szolovits, P., Pauker, S.G. 1979. Computers and clinical decision making: whether, how much, and for whom? *Proceedings of the IEEE* 67:1224–6.

Tamersoy, A., Loukides, G., Nergiz, M.E., Saygin, Y., Malin, B. 2012. Anonymization of longitudinal electronic medical records. *IEEE Transactions on Information Technology in Biomedicine* 16:413–23.

Tait, I. 1981. History of our records. *British Medical Journal* 282:702–4.

Tang, P.C., Ashe, J.S., Bates, D.W., Overhage, J.M., Sands, D.Z. 2006. Personal health records: definitions, benefits, and strategies for overcoming barriers to adoption. *Journal of the American Medical Informatics Association* 13(2):121–6.

Tassey, G. 2000. Standardization in technology-based markets. *Research Policy* 29(4–5):587–602.

Tenke, P., Köves, B., Johansen, T.E. 2014. An update on prevention and treatment of catheter-associated urinary tract infections. *Current Opinion in Infectious Diseases* 27(1):102–7.

Thielke, S., Hammond, K., Helbig, S. 2007. Copying and pasting of examinations within the electronic medical record. *International Journal of Medical Informatics* 76S:122–8.

Treloar, D., Hawayek, J., Montgomery, J.R., Russell, W., Medical Readiness Trainer Team. 2001. On-site and distance education of emergency medicine personnel with a human patient simulator. *Military Medicine* 166(11):1003–6.

Turkle, S. 2010. In good company? On the threshold of robotic companions. In Wilks, Y., ed., *Close Engagements with Artificial Companions: Key Social, Psychological, Ethical and Design Issues*. Amsterdam: John Benjamins, 3–10.

Turvey, C., Klein, D., Fix, G., Hogan, T.P., Woods, S., Simon, S.R., Charlton, M., Vaughan-Sarrazin, M., Zulman, D.M., Dindo, L., Wakefield, B., Graham, G., Nazi, K. 2014. Blue Button use by patients to access and share health record information using the Department of Veterans Affairs' online patient portal. *Journal of the American Medical Informatics Association* 21(4):657–63.

University of Toronto Joint Centre for Bioethics. 2005. *Stand On Guard for Thee: Ethical Considerations in Preparedness Planning for Pandemic Influenza*. Pandemic Influenza Working Group, Toronto: University of Toronto Joint Centre for Bioethics, available at www.jcb.utoronto.ca/people/documents/upshur_stand_guard.pdf.

Upadhyay, D.K., Sittig, D.F., Singh, H. 2014. Ebola US Patient Zero: lessons on misdiagnosis and effective use of electronic health records. *Diagnosis*, October. Epub ahead of print, DOI:10.1515/dx-2014-0064.

Urban, S. 2010. The electronic health record and the death of diagnosis. *Texas Internist*, Summer 2010, available at www.txacp.org/i4a/pages/index.cfm?pageID=876.

Urbanski, B.L., Lazenby, M. 2012. Distress among hospitalized pediatric cancer patients modified by pet-therapy intervention to improve quality of life. *Journal of Pediatric Oncology Nursing* 29(5):272–82.

US Department of Health, Education and Welfare. 1973. Records, Computers and the Rights of Citizens. (Report of the Secretary's Advisory Committee on Automated Personal Data Systems [OS]73–94.) Washington, DC: US Department of Health, Education and Welfare, available at www.justice.gov/opcl/docs/rec-com-rights.pdf and www.epic.org/privacy/hew1973report/.

van den Berge, K., Mamede, S. 2013. Cognitive diagnostic error in internal medicine. *European Journal of Internal Medicine* 24(6):525–9

Vandenbroucke, J.P. 1998. Medical journals and the shaping of medical knowledge. *The Lancet* 352:2001–6.

van der Sijs, H., Aarts, J., Vulto, A., Berg, M. 2006. Overriding of drug safety alerts in computerized physician order entry. *Journal of the American Medical Informatics Association* 13(2):138–47.

Ventres, W.B., Frankel, R.M. 2010. Patient-centered care and electronic health records: it's still about the relationship. *Family Medicine* 42(5):364–6.

Verma, I.M. 2014. Editorial expression of concern: Experimental evidence of massive-scale emotional contagion through social networks. *Proceedings of the National Academy of Sciences* 111(29):10779.

von Muhlen, M., Ohno-Machado, L. 2012. Reviewing social media use by clinicians. *Journal of the American Medical Informatics Association* 19(5):777–81.

Wachter, R. 2010. Why diagnostic errors don't get any respect – And what can be done about them. *Health Affairs* 29:1605–10.

Walker, J., Leveille, S.G., Ngo, L., Vodicka, E., Darer, J.D., Dhanireddy, S., Elmore, J.G., Feldman, H.J., Lichtenfeld, M.J., Oster, N., Ralston, J.D., Ross, S.E., Delbanco, T. 2011. Inviting patients to read their doctors' notes: patients and doctors look ahead: patient and physician surveys. *Annals of Internal Medicine* 155(12):811–9.

Walsh, C., Siegler, E.L., Cheston, E., O'Donnell, H., Collins, S., Stein, D., Vawdrey, D.K., Stetson, P.D., Informatics Intervention Research Collaboration (I2RC). 2013. Provider-to-provider electronic communication in the era of meaningful use: a review of the evidence. *Journal of Hospital Medicine* 8(10):589–97.

Wang, W,. Baggerly, K.A., Knudsen, S., Askaa, J., Mazin, W., Coombes, K.R. 2013. Independent validation of a model using cell line chemosensitivity to predict response to therapy. *Journal of the National Cancer Institute* 105(17):1284–91.

Ward, J.J., Wattier, B.A. 2011. Technology for enhancing chest auscultation in clinical simulation. *Respiratory Care* 56(6):834–45.

Warren, S.D., Brandeis, L.D. 1890. The right to privacy. *Harvard Law Review* 4(5):193–221.

Wears, R.L. 2008. The chart is dead—long live the chart. *Annals of Emergency Medicine* 52 (4):390–1.

Wears, R.L. 2015. Health information technology and victory. *Annals of Emergency Medicine* 65(2):143–5.

Weinberg, F. 1993. The history of the stethoscope. *Canadian Family Physician* 39:2223–4.

Weis, J.M., Levy, P.C. 2014. Copy, paste, and cloned notes in electronic health records: prevalence, benefits, risks, and best practice recommendations. *Chest* 145(3):632–8.

Were, M.C., Nyandiko, W.M., Huang, K.T., Slaven, J.E., Shen, C., Tierney, W.M., Vreeman, R.C. 2013. Computer-generated reminders and quality of pediatric HIV care in a resource-limited setting. *Pediatrics* 131 (3):e789–96.

Were, M.C., Shen, C., Tierney, W.M., Mamlin, J.J., Biondich, P.G., Li, X., Kimaiyo, S., Mamlin, B.W. 2011. Evaluation of computer-generated reminders to improve CD4 laboratory monitoring in sub-Saharan Africa: a prospective comparative study. *Journal of the American Medical Informatics Association* 18(2):150–5.

Whiting-O'Keefe, Q.E., Simborg, D.W., Epstein, W.V., Warger, A. 1985. A computerized summary medical record system can provide more information than the standard medical record. *Journal of the American Medical Association* 254(9):1185–92.

Wilbanks, J. 2014. Portable approaches to informed consent and open data. In Lane, J., Stodden, V., Bender, S., Nissenbaum, H., eds., *Privacy, Big Data, and the Public Good*. New York: Cambridge University Press, 235–52.

Wilks, Y. 2007. Is There Progress on Talking Sensibly to Machines? *Science* 318:927–8.

Wilks, Y., Fass, D., Guo, C.M., McDonald, J., Plate, T., Slator, B. 1990. A tractable machine dictionary as a basis for computational semantics. *Machine Translation* 5:99–154.

Williams, H., Spencer, K., Sanders, C., Lund, D., Whitley, E.A., Kaye, J., Dixon, W.G. 2015. Dynamic consent: a possible solution to improve patient confidence and trust in how electronic patient records are used in medical research. *JMIR Medical Informatics* 3(1):e3.

Williams, R., Bunduchi, R., Gerst, M., Graham, I., Pollock, N., Procter, R.N., Voss, A. 2004. Understanding the evolution of standards : alignment and reconfiguration in standards development and implementation arenas. In *Proceedings Society for Social Studies of Science (4S) & European Association for the Study of Science and Technology (EASST) conference*, Paris, August 24–28, 2004, 1–16.

Wilson, G., Aruliah, D.A., Brown, C.T., Chue Hong, N.P., Davis, M., Guy, R.T., Haddock, S.H.D., Huff, K.D., Mitchell, I. M., Plumbley, M.D., Waugh, B., White, E. P., Wilson, P. 2014. Best practices for scientific computing. *PLoS Biology* 12(1): e1001745.

Winkelstein, P. 2013. Medicine 2.0. ethical challenges of social media for the health profession. In George, C., Whitehouse, D., Duquenoy, P., eds. *eHealth: Legal, Ethical and Governance Challenges*. Heidelberg: Springer, 227–43.

Winner, L. 1980. Do artifacts have politics? *Daedalus* 109(1):121–36.

Wolf, S.M. 2013. Return of individual research results and incidental findings: facing the challenges of translational science. *Annual Review of Genomics and Human Genetics* 14:557–77.

World Health Organization. 2010. *International Statistical Classification of Diseases and Related Health Problems*. 10th Revision, Vol. 2, Instruction Manual. Geneva: World Health Organization, available at www.who.int/classifications/icd/ICD10Volume2_en_2010.pdf?ua=1.

World Health Organization. 2011. Safety and security on the Internet: Challenges and advances in Member States. Global Observatory for eHealth series – Volume 4, available at www.who.int/goe/publications/goe_security_web.pdf.

World Health Organization. 2014. Governing principles for a .health top-level domain, May 15, 2014, available at www.who.int/eheal th/ programmes/governance/en/index3.html.

Yakupcin, J.P. 2005. Child passenger safety in the school-age population. *Pediatric Emergency Care* 21(4):286–90.

Yarborough, M. 2014. Taking steps to increase the trustworthiness of scientific research. *The FASEB Journal* 28:3841–6.

Yarborough, M., Hunter, L. 2013. Teaching research ethics better: focus on excellent science, not bad scientists. *Clinical and Translational Science* 6(3):201–3.

You, J. 2015. DARPA sets out to automate research. *Science* 347(6221):465.

Youngner, S.J. 1988. Who defines futility? *Journal of the American. Medical Association* 260:2094–95.

Yu, A.C. 2006. Methods in biomedical ontology. *Journal of Biomedical Informatics* 39(3):252–66.

Zittrain, J. 2014. No, Barack Obama isn't handing control of the Internet over to China: The misguided freakout over ICANN. *The New Republic*, March 24, 2014, available at www.newrepublic.com/article/117093/us-withdraws-icann-why-its-no-big-deal.

Index

Printed in the United States
By Bookmasters